MR-Guided Focused Ultrasound

Editors

DHEERAJ GANDHI
GRAEME F. WOODWORTH

MAGNETIC RESONANCE IMAGING CLINICS OF NORTH AMERICA

www.mri.theclinics.com

Consulting Editors
SURESH K. MUKHERJI
JENNY T. BENCARDINO

November 2024 • Volume 32 • Number 4

ELSEVIER

1600 John F. Kennedy Boulevard ● Suite 1800 ● Philadelphia, Pennsylvania, 19103-2899

http://www.mri.theclinics.com

MAGNETIC RESONANCE IMAGING CLINICS OF NORTH AMERICA Volume 32, Number 4
November 2024 ISSN 1064-9689, ISBN 13: 978-0-443-24666-1

Editor: John Vassallo (j.vassallo@elsevier.com)
Developmental Editor: Sukirti Singh

Magnetic Resonance Imaging Clinics of North America (ISSN 1064-9689) is published quarterly by Elsevier Inc., 360 Park Avenue South, New York, NY 10010-1710. Months of issue are February, May, August, and November. Business and Editorial Offices: 1600 John F. Kennedy Blvd., Ste. 1800, Philadelphia, PA 19103-2899. Customer Service Office: 3251 Riverport Lane, Maryland Heights, MO 63043. Periodicals postage paid at New York, NY and additional mailing offices. Subscription prices are $420.00 per year (domestic individuals), $100.00 per year (domestic students/residents), $455.00 per year (Canadian individuals), $579.00 per year (international individuals), $100.00 per year (Canadian students/residents), and $275.00 per year (international students/residents). For institutional access pricing please contact Customer Service via the contact information below. International air speed delivery is included in all *Clinics* subscription prices. All prices are subject to change without notice. Orders, claims, and journal inquiries: Please visit our Support Hub page https://service.elsevier.com for assistance.

Reprints. For copies of 100 or more of articles in this publication, please contact the Commercial Reprints Department, Elsevier Inc., 360 Park Avenue South, New York, NY 10010-1710. Tel.: 212-633-3874; Fax: 212-633-3820; E-mail: reprints@elsevier.com.

Magnetic Resonance Imaging Clinics of North America is covered in the *RSNA Index of Imaging Literature, MEDLINE/PubMed (Index Medicus),* and *EMBASE/Excerpta Medica.*

Contributors

CONSULTING EDITORS

SURESH K. MUKHERJI, MD, MBA, FACR
Professor of Radiology and Radiation
Oncology, University of Louisville, Peoria,
Illinois, USA; Robert Wood Johnson Medical
School, Rutgers University, New Brunswick,
New Jersey, USA; Faculty, Otolaryngology
Head Neck Surgery, Michigan State University,
Farmington Hills, Michigan, USA; National

Director of Head and Neck Radiology, ProScan
Imaging, Carmel, Indiana, USA

JENNY T. BENCARDINO, MD
Vice Chair of Academic Affairs, Department of
Radiology, Montefiore Medical Center, Bronx,
New York, USA

EDITORS

DHEERAJ GANDHI, MD, FACR
Professor, Vice Chair, Departments of
Neurosurgery, Radiology and Neurology,
University of Maryland School of Medicine,
Director, Division of Neurointerventional
Surgery, Department of Diagnostic Radiology,
University of Maryland School of Medicine,
Baltimore, Maryland, USA

GRAEME F. WOODWORTH, MD, FACS
Howard M. Eisenberg Distinguished Professor
and Chair of Neurosurgery, Professor of
Radiology, Professor and Chairman,
Department of Neurosurgery, University of
Maryland School of Medicine, University of
Maryland Marlene and Stewart Greenebaum
Comprehensive Cancer Center, Baltimore,
Maryland, USA

AUTHORS

TIMOUR ABDUHALIKOV, BS
University of Virginia School of
Medicine, Charlottesville, Virginia,
USA

ABDUL-KAREEM AHMED, MD
Resident, Department of Neurosurgery,
University of Maryland School of Medicine,
Baltimore, Maryland, USA

PAVLOS ANASTASIADIS, PhD
Assistant Professor, Department of
Neurosurgery, University of Maryland
School of Medicine, University of Maryland
Marlene and Stewart Greenebaum
Comprehensive Cancer Center, Baltimore,
Maryland, USA

MARTIJN F. BOOMSMA, MD, PhD
Department of Radiology, Isala Hospital,
Imaging and Oncology Division, Image
Sciences Institute, University Medical Center
Utrecht, Utrecht, the Netherlands

DAVID R. BRENIN, MD
Co-director Focused Ultrasound Cancer
Immunotherapy Center, University of Virginia,
M.C. Wilhelm Professor, Division of Surgical
Oncology, University of Virginia Health System,
Charlottesville, Virginia, USA

JEFFREY S. CARPENTER, MD
Professor and Associate Chair, Departments
of Neuroradiology, Neuroscience, and
Neurosurgery, Rockefeller Neuroscience
Institute, West Virginia University,
Morgantown, West Virginia, USA

HUANWEN CHEN, MD
Research Fellow, National Institute of
Neurological Disorders and Stroke, National
Institutes of Health, Bethesda, Maryland, USA

MARCO COLASURDO, MD
Assistant Professor, Department of
Interventional Radiology, Oregon Health
and Science University, Portland, Oregon, USA

ZEHRA E.F. DEMIR, BS
Graduate Research Assistant, Department of
Biomedical Engineering, University of Virginia,
Charlottesville, Virginia, USA

MATTHEW DeWITT, PhD
Senior Scientist, Department of Biomedical
Engineering, Focused Ultrasound Cancer
Immunotherapy Center, University of Virginia,
Charlottesville, Virginia, USA

DHEERAJ GANDHI, MD, FACR
Professor, Vice Chair, Departments of
Neurosurgery, Radiology and Neurology,
University of Maryland School of Medicine,
Director, Division of Neurointerventional
Surgery, Department of Diagnostic Radiology,
University of Maryland School of Medicine,
Baltimore, Maryland, USA

SANGEET GHAI, MD
Associate Professor, Joint Department of
Medical Imaging, University Health Network -
Mount Sinai Hospital – Women's, College
Hospital, University of Toronto, Toronto,
Ontario, Canada

MARTIN GREEN, BS
Medical Student, East Carolina University,
Greenville, North Carolina, USA

DAYTON P. GROGAN, MD
Resident, Department of Neurosurgery,
University of Virginia Hospital, Charlottesville,
Virginia, USA

MARC W. HAUT, PhD
Professor Director of Memory Health Clinic,
Departments of Behavioral Medicine and
Psychiatry, Neurology, Neuroscience,
Rockefeller Neuroscience Institute, West Virginia
University, Morgantown, West Virginia, USA

NEAL F. KASSELL, MD
Chairman of the Focused Ultrasound
Foundation, Charlottesville, Virginia, USA

ELISABETH R. KNORREN, MD
Departments of Radiology, and Obstetrics and
Gynecology, Isala Hospital, Zwolle, the
Netherlands

VIBHOR KRISHNA, MD, SM, FACS
Associate Professor, Department of
Neurosurgery, University of North Carolina,
Chapel Hill, North Carolina, USA

NIR LIPSMAN, MD, PhD
Associate Professor, Division of Neurosurgery,
Harquail Centre for Neuromodulation,
Sunnybrook Health Sciences Centre, University
of Toronto, Toronto, Ontario, Canada

RASHI I. MEHTA, MD
Professor and Director of Cognitive
Neuroimaging, Departments of Neuroradiology,
and Neuroscience, Rockefeller Neuroscience
Institute, West Virginia University, Morgantown,
West Virginia, USA

YING MENG, MD
Neurosurgeon, Division of Neurosurgery,
Harquail Centre for Neuromodulation,
Sunnybrook Health Sciences Centre, University
of Toronto, Toronto, Ontario, Canada

SHAYAN MOOSA, MD
Assistant Professor of Neurological Surgery,
Department of Neurosurgery, University of
Virginia Hospital, Charlottesville, Virginia, USA

VANESSA MURAD, MD
Radiologist, Joint Department of Medical
Imaging, University Health Network - Mount
Sinai Hospital – Women's, College Hospital,
University of Toronto, Toronto, Ontario, Canada

INGRID M. NIJHOLT, PhD
Department of Radiology, Isala Hospital,
Zwolle, the Netherlands

NATHAN PERLIS, MD, MSC, FRCSC
Assistant Professor, Division of Urology,
Department of Surgical Oncology, University
Health Network, University of Toronto,
Toronto, Ontario, Canada

CHRISTOPHER B. POPLE, MSc
Doctoral Student and Lab Manager, Harquail
Centre for Neuromodulation, Sunnybrook
Health Sciences Centre, University of Toronto,
Toronto, Ontario, Canada

MANISH RANJAN, MBBS
Clinical Research Instructor, Department of
Neurosurgery, Rockefeller Neuroscience
Institute, West Virginia University,
Morgantown, West Virginia, USA

ALI R. REZAI, MD
Executive Chair, Departments of Neuroscience
and Neurosurgery, Rockefeller Neuroscience
Institute, West Virginia University,
Morgantown, West Virginia, USA

DANIEL ROQUE, MD
Director, UNC Movement Disorders
Neuromodulation Program, Associate
Professor, Movement Disorders, Department
of Neurology, University of North Carolina,
Chapel Hill, North Carolina, USA

JOKE M. SCHUTTE, MD, PhD
Department of Obstetrics and Gynecology,
Isala Hospital, Zwolle, the Netherlands

THOMAS SHERLOCK, BS
Graduate Research Assistant, Department of
Biomedical Engineering, University of Virginia,
Charlottesville, Virginia, USA

NATASHA D. SHEYBANI, PhD
Assistant Professor, Department of Biomedical
Engineering, Focused Ultrasound Cancer
Immunotherapy Center, University of Virginia,
Department of Radiology and Medical Imaging,
University of Virginia, Charlottesville, Virginia,
USA

NICOLE SILVA, MD
Resident Physician, Department of
Neurosurgery, University of North Carolina,
Chapel Hill, North Carolina, USA

CHRISTIN A. TIEGS-HEIDEN, MD
Associate Professor of Radiology, Division of
Musculoskeletal Radiology, Mayo Clinic,
Rochester, Minnesota, USA

GRAEME F. WOODWORTH, MD, FACS
Howard M. Eisenberg Distinguished Professor
and Chair of Neurosurgery, Professor of
Radiology, Professor and Chairman,
Department of Neurosurgery, University of
Maryland School of Medicine, University of
Maryland Marlene and Stewart Greenebaum
Comprehensive Cancer Center, Baltimore,
Maryland, USA

Contents

Transcranial Focused Ultrasound: A History of Our Future   585

Abdul-Kareem Ahmed, Graeme F. Woodworth, and Dheeraj Gandhi

The history of focused ultrasound is a parallel history of neuroradiology, functional neurosurgery, and physics and engineering. Multiple pioneers collaborated as ultrasound transitioned from a wartime technology to a therapeutic one, particularly in using it to ablate the brain to treat movement disorders. Several competing technologies ensured that this "ultrasonic neurosurgery" remained in a lull. An algorithm and other advancements that obviated a craniectomy for ultrasonic neurosurgery allowed magnetic resonance-guided focused ultrasound to flourish to its modern phase.

MR Imaging-Guided Focused Ultrasound for Breast Tumors   593

Matthew DeWitt, Zehra E.F. Demir, Thomas Sherlock, David R. Brenin, and Natasha D. Sheybani

Breast tumors remain a complex and prevalent health burden impacting millions of individuals worldwide. Challenges in treatment arise from the invasive nature of traditional surgery and, in malignancies, the complexity of treating metastatic disease. The development of noninvasive treatment alternatives is critical for improving patient outcomes and quality of life. This review aims to explore the advancements and applications of focused ultrasound (FUS) technology over the past 2 decades. FUS offers a promising noninvasive, nonionizing intervention strategy in breast tumors including primary breast cancer, fibroadenomas, and metastatic breast cancer.

Magnetic Resonance–Guided Focused Ultrasound Surgery for Gynecologic Indications   615

Elisabeth R. Knorren, Ingrid M. Nijholt, Joke M. Schutte, and Martijn F. Boomsma

Magnetic resonance–guided focused ultrasound surgery (MRgFUS) appears to be an effective and safe treatment for uterine fibroids and adenomyosis, particularly in women who wish to preserve fertility. In abdominal wall endometriosis and painful recurrent gynecologic malignances, MRgFUS can relieve pain, but more research is needed. There is no widespread reimbursement due to the lack of large prospective or randomized controlled trials comparing MRgFUS with standard therapy.

Prostate cancer (PCa) is a prevalent malignancy in men, and the management of lo-calized disease has evolved significantly in recent years. Focal therapy, wherein the biopsy confirmed site of tumor with margins is treated leaving the remaining gland intact, has emerged as a promising strategy for treating localized clinically significant PCa, minimizing side effects associated with radical therapies. We present the tech-nical aspects, a summary of the most relevant evidence to date on the performance and safety of this technique, and the characteristic MR imaging findings during treat-ment, in the early posttreatment period and in the long term.

MR-guided focused ultrasound (MRgFUS) has a wide range of musculoskeletal ap-plications. Some indications are well validated, specifically the treatment of painful osseous metastases and osteoid osteoma. Others are only beginning to be studied, such as the treatment of painful facet, sacroiliac, and knee joints. MRgFUS of soft tissue lesions also shows promise, particularly in patients whom alternative modal-ities are not feasible or may result in significant morbidity. Ongoing and future re-search will illuminate the full potential for MRgFUS in the treatment of musculoskeletal conditions.

Focused ultrasound ablation achieves selective thermal lesioning of the thalamic and basal ganglia targets using real-time MR imaging guidance. It is US Food and Drug Administration-approved to treat essential tremor and Parkinson's disease tremor, fluctuations, and dyskinesias. Patients often seek focused ultrasound treat-ment because symptom relief is immediate, and hardware implantation is not re-quired. This review summarizes the current and potential future application of focused ultrasound ablation to treat movement disorders. We also discuss the on-going research optimizing the technique of focused ultrasound ablation to improve long-term efficacy and minimize the risk of side effects.

MR-guided focused ultrasound (FUS) represents a promising alternative for patients with chronic neuropathic who have failed medical management and other treatment options. Early single-center experience with chronic neuropathic pain and trigeminal neuralgia has demonstrated favorable long-term outcomes. Excellent safety profile with low risk of motor and sensory complications and so far anecdotal permanent neurologic deficits make FUS a powerful tool to treat patients who are otherwise hopeless. Neuromodulation may be the most influential factor driving outcomes and studies devised to detect neuroplasticity will be critical to guide such therapies.

Malignant gliomas (MGs) are the most common primary brain tumors in adults. Despite recent advances in understanding the biology and potential therapeutic vulnerabilities of MGs, treatment options remain limited as the delivery of drugs is often impeded by the blood-brain barrier (BBB), and safe, complete surgical resection may not always be possible, especially for deep-seated tumors. In this review, the authors highlight emerging applications for MR imaging–guided focused ultrasound (MRgFUS) as a noninvasive treatment modality for MGs. Specifically, the authors discuss MRgFUS's potential role in direct tumor cell killing, opening the BBB, and modulating antitumor immunity.

Neurodegenerative diseases are a leading cause of death and disability and pose a looming global public health crisis. Despite progress in understanding biological and molecular factors associated with these disorders and their progression, effective disease modifying treatments are presently limited. Focused ultrasound (FUS) is an emerging therapeutic strategy for Alzheimer's disease, Parkinson's disease, and amyotrophic lateral sclerosis. In these contexts, applications of FUS include neuroablation, neuromodulation, and/or blood-brain barrier opening with and without facilitated intracerebral drug delivery. Here, the authors review preclinical evidence and current and emerging applications of FUS for neurodegenerative diseases and summarize future directions in the field.

Breakthroughs in medical imaging and ultrasound transducer design have led to feasible application of focused ultrasound (FUS) to intracranial pathologies. Currently, one of the most active fields in FUS has been the temporary disruption the blood–brain barrier. In addition to enhancing drug delivery to the brain, FUS blood–brain barrier disruption may allow liberation of biomarkers from the brain, thus facilitating ease of detection and adding the element of spatial specificity to an otherwise nonspecific test. This study reviews the current evidence to support FUS liquid biopsy and the challenges of advancing this field.

MR-guided focused ultrasound (MRgFUS) allows for the incisionless treatment of intracranial lesions in an outpatient setting. While this is currently approved for the surgical treatment of essential tremor and Parkinson's disease, advancements in imaging and ultrasound technology are allowing for the expansion of treatment indications to other intracranial diseases. In addition, these advancements are also making MRgFUS treatments easier, safer, and more efficacious.

MAGNETIC RESONANCE IMAGING CLINICS OF NORTH AMERICA

SERIES OF RELATED INTEREST

Advances in Clinical Radiology
www.advancesinclinicalradiology.com
Neuroimaging Clinics
www.neuroimaging.theclinics.com
PET Clinics
www.pet.theclinics.com
Radiologic Clinics
www.radiologic.theclinics.com

VISIT THE CLINICS ONLINE!
Access your subscription at:
www.theclinics.com

JOURNAL TITLE: Magnetic Resonance Imaging Clinics of North America

ISSUE: 32.4

PROGRAM OBJECTIVE

The goal of *Magnetic Resonance Imaging Clinics of North America* is to keep practicing physicians up to date with current clinical practice by providing timely articles reviewing the state of the art in patient care.

TARGET AUDIENCE

All practicing physicians and healthcare professionals who provide patient care utilizing findings from Magnetic Resonance Imaging.

LEARNING OBJECTIVES

Upon completion of this activity, participants will be able to:

1. Review advantages of magnetic resonance imaging (MRI)-guided focused ultrasound (MRgFUS).
2. Discuss magnetic resonance imaging-guided focused ultrasound (MRgFUS) as an emerging non-invasive technology for managing brain tumors.
3. Recognize that focused ultrasound (FUS) offers a promising non-invasive and non-ionizing intervention strategy in various medical diagnoses, including primary breast cancer.

ACCREDITATION

The Elsevier Office of Continuing Medical Education (EOCME) is accredited by the Accreditation Council for Continuing Medical Education (ACCME) to provide continuing medical education for physicians.

The EOCME designates this journal-based CME activity enduring material for a maximum of 11 *AMA PRA Category 1 Credit*(s)™. Physicians should claim only the credit commensurate with the extent of their participation in the activity.

All other healthcare professionals requesting continuing education credit for this enduring material will be issued a certificate of participation.

DISCLOSURE OF RELEVANT FINANCIAL RELATIONSHIPS

The EOCME evaluates the relevancy of financial relationships with its instructors, faculty, planners, and other individuals who are in a position to control the content of CME activities. The EOCME will review all identified disclosures and mitigate financial relationships with ineligible companies, as applicable. An ineligible company is any entity whose primary business is producing, marketing, selling, re-selling, or distributing healthcare products used by or on patients. For specific examples of ineligible companies visit accme.org/standards. EOCME is committed to providing its learners with CME activities that promote improvements or quality in healthcare and not a specific proprietary business or a commercial interest.

The authors and editors listed below have identified no financial relationships or relationships to products or devices they have with ineligible companies related to the content of this CME activity:
Timour Abduhalikov, BS; Abdul-Kareem Ahmed, MD; Pavlos Anastasiadis, PhD; Martijn F. Boomsma, MD, PhD; David R. Brenin, MD; Jeffrey S. Carpenter, MD; Huanwen Chen, MD; Marco Colasurdo, MD; Zehra E.F. Demir; Matthew DeWitt, PhD; Martin Green, BS; Dayton P. Grogan, MD; Marc W. Haut, PhD; Neal F. Kassell, MD; Loes R. Knorren; Vibhor Krishna, MD; Nir Lipsman, MD, PhD; Rashi I. Mehta, MD; Ying Meng, MD; Shayan Moosa, MD; Vanessa Murad, MD; Ingrid M. Nijholt, PhD; Nathan Perlis, MD, MSc, FRCSC; Christopher Pople, MS; Manish Ranjan, MBBS; Ali R. Rezai, MD; Daniel Roque, MD; Joke M. Schutte, MD, PhD; Thomas Sherlock; Natasha D. Sheybani, PhD; Nicole Silva, MD; Christin A. Tiegs-Heiden, MD; John Vassallo; Graeme F. Woodworth, MD, FACS

The authors and editors listed below have identified financial relationships or relationships to products or devices they have with ineligible companies related to the content of this CME activity:
Dheeraj Gandhi, MD: Researcher: MircroVention Inc., NoNo Inc.

Sangeet Ghai, MD: Researcher: Insightec

The Clinics staff listed below have identified no financial relationships or relationships to products or devices they have with ineligible companies related to the content of this CME activity:
Kothainayaki Kulanthaivelu; Michelle Littlejohn; Patrick J. Manley; Malvika Shah; John Vassallo

UNAPPROVED/OFF-LABEL USE DISCLOSURE

The EOCME requires CME faculty to disclose to the participants:

1. When products or procedures being discussed are off-label, unlabelled, experimental, and/or investigational (not US Food and Drug Administration [FDA] approved); and
2. Any limitations on the information presented, such as data that are preliminary or that represent ongoing research, interim analyses, and/or unsupported opinions. Faculty may discuss information about pharmaceutical agents that is outside of FDA-approved labelling. This information is intended solely for CME and is not intended to promote off-label use of these

medications. If you have any questions, contact the medical affairs department of the manufacturer for the most recent prescribing information.

TO ENROLL

To enroll in the *Magnetic Resonance Imaging Clinics of North America* Continuing Medical Education program, call customer service at 1-800-654-2452 or sign up online at http://www.theclinics.com/home/cme. The CME program is available to subscribers for an additional annual fee of USD 270.00.

METHOD OF PARTICIPATION

In order to claim credit, participants must complete the following:
1. Complete enrolment as indicated above.
2. Read the activity.
3. Complete the CME Test and Evaluation. Participants must achieve a score of 70% on the test. All CME Tests and Evaluations must be completed online.

CME INQUIRIES/SPECIAL NEEDS

For all CME inquiries or special needs, please contact elsevierCME@elsevier.com.

Foreword
MR-Guided Focused Ultrasound

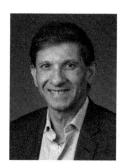 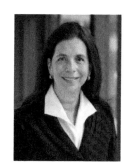

Suresh K. Mukherji, MD, MBA, FACR   Jenny T. Bencardino, MD

Consulting Editors

MR-guided focused ultrasound (MRgFUS) is an important noninvasive treatment technique with numerous FDA-approved indications. These include treatment of uterine fibroids, various prostate disorders, painful bone metastasis, osteoid osteoma, liver tumors (histotripsy), and various neurologic diseases, which include essential tremors, tremor-dominant Parkinson disease, and Parkinson dyskinesia.

The recent expansion of approved indications was why we invited Drs Dheeraj Gandhi and Graeme Woodworth to guest edit an issue of *Magnetic Resonance Imaging Clinics of North America* devoted to MRgFUS. This edition provides an overview of the current clinical applications of this important minimally invasive technique. This issue contains eleven articles starting with the history of MRgFUS followed by articles devoted to current applications for treating a variety of breast, musculoskeletal, gynecology, prostate, neuro-oncology, and neurodegenerative disorders.

I would like to thank all the coauthors for their wonderful contributions. The articles are concise and comprehensive state-of-the-art review articles that cover a broad range of topics. I would like to thank Drs Gandhi and Woodworth for guest editing this magnificent issue, which will serve as

an important reference for MRgFUS for many years to come. On a personal note, Dr Gandhi was one of the most talented neuroradiology fellows I (SKM) ever trained; I also had the privilege of working with him for several years before he was eventually recruited to University of Maryland, where he is currently Professor and Chief of Neurointerventional Radiology and Vice Chair of Academic Affairs. It is my pleasure to continue to be his colleague and friend!

Suresh K. Mukherji, MD, MBA, FACR
University of Louisville &
University of Illinois
ProScan Imaging
Carmel, IN 46032, USA

Jenny T. Bencardino, MD
Vice Chair of Academic Affairs
Department of Radiology
Montefiore Medical Center
111 East 210th Street
Bronx, New York 10467-2401, USA

E-mail addresses:
sureshmukherji@hotmail.com (S.K. Mukherji)
jbencardin@montefiore.org (J.T. Bencardino)

Magn Reson Imaging Clin N Am 32 (2024) xiii
https://doi.org/10.1016/j.mric.2024.06.001
1064-9689/24/© 2024 Published by Elsevier Inc.

Preface

Incisionless Precision Surgery with MR Imaging–Guided Focused Ultrasound: A Look into the Future

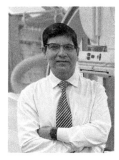 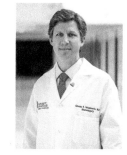

Dheeraj Gandhi, MD, FACR   Graeme F. Woodworth, MD, FACS

Editors

Whatever you can do, or dream you can, begin it. Boldness has genius, power, and magic in it.

—*Johann Wolfgang von Goethe*

The emergence of minimally invasive techniques has constituted a monumental leap forward in the rapidly evolving landscapes of surgery and neurosurgery. Traditionally, the prospect of surgery evokes images of exposed, open anatomy, prolonged hospital stays, and arduous recoveries. However, the advent of minimally invasive approaches shifts this paradigm, revolutionizing the field with techniques that prioritize precision, safety and patient well-being. Surgical procedures that can be administered in the outpatient setting are increasingly desirable, especially if the procedures can be coupled with other benefits, such as avoidance of general anesthesia, lower risk of infection, and more rapid return to daily activities. MR imaging–guided focused ultrasound (MRgFUS) presents many of these advantages, along with the addition of being incisionless, having high temporospatial precision, and enabling real-time patient and treatment feedback.

This issue of *Magnetic Resonance Imaging Clinics of North America* is an effort to provide the readers with an overview of MRgFUS starting with its fascinating history of development followed by state-of-the-art reviews describing its current applications in the breast, musculoskeletal system, gynecology, prostate as well as brain surgery. MR imaging guidance is a key feature, as it enhances the precision in treatment planning, allows real-time thermal, susceptibility, and/or acoustic resonance feedback monitoring and thereby enables highly controlled, prescriptive, and conformal therapies.[1,2] Moreover, it allows for intraoperative and postoperative imaging in the same setting.

At the time of this publication, the FDA has already approved nine indications for focused ultrasound (FUS). These include the treatment of uterine fibroids, prostate diseases, benign prostatic hyperplasia, painful bone metastasis, osteoid osteoma, liver tumors (histotripsy) and neurologic applications in essential tremors, tremor-dominant Parkinson disease, and Parkinson dyskinesia. In the year 2023, FUS reached a critical milestone, crossing 100,000 patient treatments.[3] However, it is hoped that this is just the beginning of a long and fruitful journey. We need to continue to build momentum, advance and diversify technology as well as to deliver appropriate and effective FUS therapies to potentially millions of people worldwide.

Regarding mechanisms of action, FUS is a versatile tool since it can produce wide-ranging

Magn Reson Imaging Clin N Am 32 (2024) xv–xvi
https://doi.org/10.1016/j.mric.2024.04.007
1064-9689/24/

bioeffects in human tissues that can be transient, such as neuromodulation and blood-brain barrier opening, or permanent, such as thermal ablation, histotripsy, and clot lysis. Moreover, FUS can facilitate other complex alterations, such as immune cell trafficking, radiosensitization and chemosensitization, acoustic activation, and enhanced drug delivery.[1,4] These properties make FUS a unique tool that will play an increasingly significant role in the treatment of a wide array of diseases in the future. However, amid all the optimism surrounding minimally invasive surgeries with MRgFUS, it is also crucial to acknowledge the challenges that lie ahead. Regulatory considerations, technological limitations, the relatively high cost of care delivery, and the need for multidisciplinary teams are among the hurdles that must be addressed to realize the full potential of these groundbreaking techniques.

An international group of authors chosen for this endeavor are recognized for their expertise and experience with this fascinating technology. We have enjoyed working with these experts, who have contributed generously to this issue. At times, there is a slight overlap in the content that it is hoped will provide differing perspectives of physicians and researchers from varied backgrounds and institutions.

We are thankful to the Elsevier staff members: Shivank Joshi, Malvika Shah, and John Vassallo, for all their help. Many thanks to the Consulting Editor and a good friend, Suresh Mukherji, for this great honor. We hope that the readers enjoy reading these articles and be inspired to incorporate MRgFUS in their practice as well as improve access of this technology to their patients.

DISCLOSURE

D. Gandhi reports grants from Microvention, Focused Ultrasound Foundation, NIH, and University Calgary/NoNo Therapeutics. G.F. Woodworth reports grants from NIH, Focused ultrasound Foundation, and clinical trial support from Insightec and the Keep Punching Foundation.

Dheeraj Gandhi, MD, FACR
Departments of Neurosurgery
Neurology and Radiology
University of Maryland School of Medicine
22 South Green Street
Baltimore, MD 21201, USA

Graeme F. Woodworth, MD, FACS
Department of Neurosurgery and
Department of Radiology
University of Maryland School of Medicine
22 South Green Street
Baltimore, MD 21201, USA

E-mail addresses:
dgandhi@umm.edu (D. Gandhi)
gwoodworth@som.umaryland.edu
(G.F. Woodworth)

REFERENCES

1. Anastasiadis P, Gandhi D, Guo Y, et al. Localized blood-brain barrier opening in infiltrating gliomas with MRI-guided acoustic emissions-controlled focused ultrasound. Proc Natl Acad Sci U S A 2021; 118(37):e2103280118.
2. Ahmed AK, Zhuo J, Gullapalli RP, et al. Focused ultrasound central lateral thalamotomy for the treatment of refractory neuropathic pain: phase I trial. Neurosurgery 2024;94(4):690–9.
3. Focused Ultrasound foundation: 2023 year in review report, Available at: https://cdn.fusfoundation.org/2024/04/01100027/Focused-Ultrasound-Foundation-Year-in-Review-Report-2023_March-28.pdf. Accessed: March 26, 2024.
4. Ahmed N, Gandhi D, Melhem ER, et al. MRI guided focused ultrasound-mediated delivery of therapeutic cells to the brain: a review of the state-of-the-art methodology and future applications. Front Neurol 2021; 12:669449.

Transcranial Focused Ultrasound
A History of Our Future

Abdul-Kareem Ahmed, MD[a], Graeme F. Woodworth, MD[a],
Dheeraj Gandhi, MD[a,b,c,d],*

KEYWORDS

• Functional neurosurgery • Focused ultrasound • Thalamotomy • Pallidotomy

KEY POINTS

• Ultrasound was advanced as a technology at the turn of the twentieth century, eventually transitioning from wartime use to medical applications.
• Focused ultrasound was developed by a niche group of physicists, engineers, radiologists, neurologists, and neurosurgeons to treat movement disorders; however, multiple other treatment modalities outcompeted it.
• Modern focused ultrasound came to the fore after a craniectomy was obviated, ushering in multiple trials for the treatment of neurologic and psychiatric diseases.

INTRODUCTION

Transcranial magnetic resonance-guided focused ultrasound (MRgFUS) is becoming increasingly utilized to treat a growing number of neurologic and psychiatric diseases.[1] In the United States, MRgFUS has achieved regulatory approval to treat essential tremor, tremor dominant Parkinson's disease, and dyskinesias of Parkinson's disease. Additionally, neuropathic pain, depression, Alzheimer's disease, drug delivery for glioblastoma, and obsessive compulsive disorder, along with many other indications are currently being explored in clinical trials.[2-4]

Focused ultrasound (FUS) has the potential to create varied effects, including but not limited to thermal ablation, neuromodulation, blood–brain barrier disruption, and histotripsy.[5] The earliest and most established indications utilize thermal ablation; however, neuromodulation and blood–brain barrier disruption are being fervently investigated to treat oncological, neurodegenerative, and psychiatric diseases, among others.

With the current interest in MRgFUS, and the expansion of investigation for its use, it may be useful to the research and clinical community to understand and reflect on the history of its genesis and development. As with any new technology, there are technical and regulatory challenges that MRgFUS currently faces. With a review of the history of FUS, lessons from the past may inform the path forward today. Furthermore, MRgFUS technology stands on the shoulders of those individuals who were at the cutting-edge of their respective fields, be it physics, engineering, radiology, neurology, or neurosurgery, and they deserve significant recognition.

[a] Department of Neurosurgery, University of Maryland School of Medicine, 22 South Green Street, Baltimore, MD 21201, USA; [b] Division of Neurointerventional Surgery, Department of Diagnostic Radiology, University of Maryland School of Medicine, 22 South Green Street, Baltimore, MD 21201, USA; [c] Department of Radiology, University of Maryland School of Medicine, 22 South Green Street, Baltimore, MD 21201, USA; [d] Department of Neurology, University of Maryland School of Medicine, 22 South Green Street, Baltimore, MD 21201, USA
* Corresponding author. Division of Neurointerventional Surgery, Department of Diagnostic Radiology, University of Maryland School of Medicine, 22 South Green Street, Baltimore, MD 21201.
E-mail address: dgandhi@umm.edu

Magn Reson Imaging Clin N Am 32 (2024) 585–592
https://doi.org/10.1016/j.mric.2024.04.002
1064-9689/24/© 2024 Elsevier Inc. All rights reserved.

A SONIC BOON

The history of FUS begins with the development of ultrasound itself. Ultrasound technology has its basis in piezoelectricity or the reverse piezoelectric effect. Particular crystalline structures like quartz produce electrical charge when pressure is applied to them, the piezoelectric effect, a phenomenon which was first reported by brothers and physicists Jacques and Pierre Curie in 1880.[6] The reverse is also true, some crystalline structures will change shape when subject to electrical force, which was mathematically proven by physicist Gabriel Lippmann and confirmed by the Curie brothers the following year.[7,8] Therefore, electrical current passed through quartz could cause it to vibrate, producing sound.

In a delayed manner, this discovery gave way to industrial, military, and medical applications.[9]

At the turn of the century, the exploration of echolocation was spurred by significant events such as the 1912 sinking of the RMS *Titanic* and the onset of World War I. In response to these catalysts, physicist Paul Langevin and engineer Constantin Chilowski collaborated to pioneer underwater ultrasonic echolocation, a breakthrough that would prove indispensable for submarine navigation and the detection of German U-boats.[10] This early form of sonar technology marked a pivotal moment in maritime warfare, laying the foundation for subsequent advancements that would play a critical role in shaping the outcome of conflicts.

In parallel, medical applications were being explored. Quartz and ceramics could be used to produce ultrasound for diagnostic or therapeutic purposes.[11] The first use of ultrasound for imaging purposes was with the through-transmission method, wherein Austrian neurologist Karl Dussik placed transducers on both sides of a patient's partially submerged head to try to image his ventricles.[12,13] The result was mostly artifact due to reflections and attenuations from the skull, the first signs of a lasting conundrum, but a different method, pulse-echo, followed and succeeded.[14,15] With pulse-echo, the transducer produces and receives sound waves and reflected echoes. This birthed modern diagnostic ultrasound, which is achieved with a sound frequency range of 0.5 to 30 MHz.[11]

AN EARLY CONVERGENCE

With the field of diagnostic ultrasound burgeoning, very few tinkered with ultrasound as a therapeutic modality.[16] As it relates to the topic at hand, in 1935 Johannes Gruetzmacher in Berlin was the first to consider using a curved crystal, as opposed to traditional linear ones, to converge short ultrasound waves onto a focal point, thus developing the first true "focused" ultrasound.[17] He noted, "At the convergence point, because of the accumulation effect, an extremely large amount of energy summation occurs" [German, translated].

John Lynn and Tracy Putnam built upon this study. They developed an ultrasound generator for producing focal lesions.[18] The top of this contraption was a cellophane diaphragm on which to place biological specimens. Below it, the container housing the curved crystal was filled with transformer oil, and air occupied the space behind the crystal. The team first produced lesions in paraffin blocks, then beef liver. They noted that focusing effects were most accurate when energy was applied instantaneously. In vivo experiments in animals to produce cerebral lesions proved difficult. Damage to the scalp and overlying tissues was noted due to the device's small application area, high ultrasonic frequency, and low output of the radiofrequency power source. Based on neuroanatomical location, they produced transient hind limb weakness in a dog and transient blindness in a cat.

In a follow-up report, Lynn and Putnam's ultrasonic generator had a quartz plate 5.08 cm in diameter, vibrating at a frequency of 835 kHz, with a focal point 4 cm above the cellophane diaphragm.[19] In total, they conducted in vivo experiments to produce cerebral lesions on 3 dogs, 30 cats, and 4 monkeys. A few millimeters of olive oil were used between cellophane and skin surface, making sure to reduce air bubbles as air causes dispersion and high impedance. Again, they produced transient neurologic changes but noted that skin damage would eventually result in necrosis and gangrene. Neurologic changes became permanent if a greater quantity of energy was applied. Cerebral lesions could only be produced if the overlying tissues were thin. Intervening tissue resulted in the disruption of energy focusing, a problem yet to be solved. A conical lesion of the premotor area of a monkey was noted on histologic analysis.

THE FRY BROTHERS AND RUSSELL MEYERS

During the wane of World War II, the G.I. Bill was enacted enabling veterans to further their training and education in civilian environments. Students flooded universities, and military research and development transitioned to an extent to university campuses, including the University of Illinois.[20] Engineering was a popular field of study.

Physicist William J. Fry joined the University in 1946 who, in response to the war, had previously worked at the Naval Research Laboratory in Washington, DC on sonar systems. His brother Francis J. Fry, an electrical engineer, joined his brother, from Westinghouse Electric Corp. His division was a contractor for the Manhattan Project, affording him experience in radiation research. Space was limited, so Bill and Frank settled on an unoccupied location in a steam tunnel at the University of Illinois. This was the first home of their newly established Bioacoustics Research Laboratory.

The brothers wanted to study the brain and develop a circuit-diagram of its connections. They envisioned FUS as a noninvasive method to study brain anatomy and eventually to alter it. In the early 1950s, they studied the propagation of ultrasound in tissue, how ultrasound is scattered and attenuated, particularly in nervous tissue. Funding came from the US Navy's Bureau of Ships and the Office of Naval Research.[20] Using cat and monkey models, the brothers and colleagues found that ultrasound affects tissue components differently, a threshold exists to cause permanent damage, multiple applications of ultrasound below threshold can cause transient change, and amplitude and exposure time, in part, govern these effects.[21–25]

Their study introduced "ultrasonic neurosurgery" in large part due to their novel transducer. In the mid-1950s, the Fry brothers and colleagues produced focal lesions, sometimes 2 to 3 mm wide in the animals with no damage to surrounding tissue or blood vessels.[26,27] One important clinical collaboration was with William H. Mosberg, a neurosurgeon at the University of Maryland, Baltimore.[27] The technique required performing a craniectomy. With saline as a favorable medium reducing impedance between the 4 ultrasound beams and the dura, unintended damage was minimal. Localization of the target was achieved in an elegant way. As with many tools that would eventually aid FUS development, stereotaxy was maturing in parallel.[28]

The head of the subject was first fixated in a stereotactic frame of 4 pins.[27] A radiopaque ventriculogram was then performed. The anterior commissure-posterior commissure plane was noted. In this roentgenogram, the location of the target was produced by the shadow of a retractable metal pointer, which was adjusted in space to reflect this location in vertical and longitudinal coordinates. By considering the deployed pointer's size, its location, and scaling effects, the determined location of the target in 3 dimensional space in relation to the frame was known. The tip of the deployed pointer is always the focal convergence point for the 4 beams. A few days later, after ventricular gas absorbs, the patient is repositioned into the frame with 4 pins in shallow burr holes

exactly as prior, and roentgenograms confirm position. The 4 beam ultrasound transducer is positioned as previously calculated. A craniectomy is performed in situ.

To test this setup in patients, the Fry brothers collaborated with University of Iowa neurosurgeon Russell Meyers.[29] In the 1930s and 1940s, neurosurgeons were performing destructive or ablative surgery to treat patients with Parkinson's disease, postencephalitic parkinsonism, and other movement disorders, at first targeting the pyramidal system.[30–32] Paralysis was a meager win over tremor, setting Meyers to focus on the extrapyramidal system, the first to do so.[33] At the time, Walter Dandy called the extrapyramidal system the "the center of consciousness."[34] Meyers experimented with resecting the anterior two-thirds of the caudate nucleus via a transventricular approach in a patient with parkinsonism, which resulted in lasting relief, presenting his decade-long study in 1951.[35] He continued his exploration of disrupting the basal ganglia in patients with Parkinson's disease and found that pallidofugal sectioning was most effective. In parallel, in 1952, Irving Cooper made his serendipitous discovery when during a planned pedunculotomy for parkinsonism, he accidentally ligated the anterior choroidal artery, thereby resulting in an ischemic pallidotomy, improving the patient's symptoms. He and others advanced this into the chemopallidotomy using a catheter and alcohol injection.[32] Pallidotomy and then thalamotomy began to be performed. Basal ganglia surgery became of keen interest for movement disorders; however, morbidity and mortality was high. In this brief window, before stereotaxy and other methods like electrocoagulation took the field, ultrasound lesioning with a craniectomy was an attractive alternative.

The Fry brothers and Meyers built a novel 2 floor operating room to accommodate their navigable ultrasound transducer and a full neurosurgery repertoire.[36] In a series of 12 patients with tremor and rigidity, they targeted the ansa lenticularis (980 kHz, 2.3 seconds) or the medial globus pallidus or substantia nigra (980 kHz, 3.0 seconds) (**Fig. 1**). Patients experience abolition of their tremor and rigidity depending on positioning. The success of the apparatus and surgery was featured in the December 1957 issue of *Time* magazine, noting it was "unheard, unseen, but sharper than the scalpel."[37] The team expanded their technique for more movement disorders and set their sights on ablation for neoplastic disease and psychiatric disease as well.[38] For this transient moment, it would seem "ultrasonic neurosurgery" was here to stay. But many parallel and pending discoveries were being made.

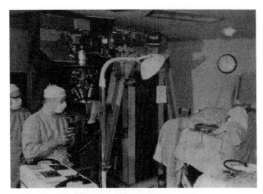

Fig. 1. Russell Meyers in a modified operating room treatment a patient with Parkinsonism featured in *Time Magazine*. (*From* Time 1957, public domain.[37])

MANY COMPETITORS

If ultrasonic neurosurgery did not become standard of care for the treatment of movement disorders and other neurologic disorders, the responsibility may be placed in one or all of the following. The prerequisite of performing a craniectomy was the main barrier, a morbid surgery for a tremor or other ailment. In addition, stereotactic methods became more precise, from Spiegel and Wycis to modern stereotaxy, eventually aided by computed tomography (CT) and MR imaging.[28,39] This allowed alternative methods to flourish. Radiofrequency ablation, lesioning using an intraparenchymal probe through a burr hole, became a simpler solution. Stereotactic radiosurgery, the discovery of levodopa, and, finally, deep brain stimulation (DBS) shelved ablative techniques, including FUS, in a corner.

In the 1940s and 1950s, with the advancement of stereotactic approaches, pallidotomy and eventually by serendipity thalamotomy were performed for Parkinsonism and other movement disorders, using catheters or cannulas to chemically or electrically destroy the target, and eventually using radiofrequency ablation.[31,32,40] Exact targeting varied by group, between the globus palludius internus (GPi), ansa lentricularis, and the ventrolateral nucleus of the thalamus. By 1960, the thalamus was preferred, but Lars Leksell and colleagues demonstrated the high success rate of targeting the posteromedial GPi.[41] Around this time, Leksell developed the first stereotactic radiosurgery, and a thalamotomy for intractable pain was his first disease target.[42] Though the effect of radiosurgery takes several months to manifest, another less invasive method to surgically treat movement disorders came to the fore.[43] FUS had little footing left.

The discovery and introduction of levodopa heralded a precipitous decline in pallidotomy and thalamotomy approaches for Parkinsonism and other movement disorders, except within a small enclave of neurosurgeons.[32] The 1960s and 1970s were the pharmacologic age. In 1957, Arvid Carlsson serendipitously discovered that reserpine-treated rabbits suffered from dopamine depletion, which was concentrated in the striatum.[44] Subsequent study by George Cotzias and others led to the logical conclusion that Parkinsonism could be modified with dopamine repletion, levodopa.[30,45,46] Unfortunately, in 5 to 7 years, most patients experienced levodopa-induced motor fluctuations. Pallidotomy could be used to relieve these dyskinesias.

The final serendipity, the lasting competitor to enter the field, was DBS. In 1987, Alim Louis Benabid and colleagues were electrically stimulating the thalamus for a planned thalamotomy for essential tremor.[47] They found that at frequencies above 100 Hz, symptoms could be immediately attenuated and modified. Further research demonstrated that this stimulation could be performed safely, bilaterally, and could be permanently implanted.[30] Today, DBS is used for essential tremor, Parkinson's disease, and dystonia and is being investigated for psychiatric disorders.[48] Surely in this time, a procedure requiring a craniectomy to ultrasonically ablate deep brain nuclei was rarely entertained.

THE ALGORITHM

A few pioneers continued to investigate transcranial FUS during this lull. In the 1970s, Robert Heimburger collaborated with Frank Fry and others to assess the utility of ultrasound for brain imaging.[49-52] In 1985, Heimburger reported 13 years of study using high-intensity FUS to thermally destroy intracranial tumors, after craniectomy, resection, and wire mesh placement, to take advantage of an acoustic window.[53] In some patients, low-intensity FUS was used to improve chemotherapeutic penetration. In a similar experiment, Norman Guthkelch, Kullervo Hynynen, and others reported in 1991 using FUS and external beam radiation for primary malignant brain tumors, through a craniectomy window.[54] Again, the intact cranium was an impenetrable problem for FUS.

In 1993, Hynynen demonstrated the feasibility of using MR imaging to monitor FUS tissue necrosis in the thigh of a greyhound, beginning the era of MR-guided FUS.[55] In 1998, Hynynen and Ferenc Jolesz performed water bath experiments, using 2 phased arrays of 64 ultrasound elements. They attempted to create focal lesions in harvested rabbit brain through an intact human skull.[56] By measuring and compensating for the phase shifts caused by the skull, a sharp focus could be achieved with pulsed sonication at 0.559 MHz. This was the pre-amble to a breakthrough. In the next year, Chrit Moonen and colleagues demonstrated utilizing MR thermometry to monitor tissue temperature of rat leg muscle during FUS sonication.[57]

In 2002, the revolution came. Gregory Clement and Hynynen reported their modern transcranial FUS method.[58] Using a 320 element hemispherical phased array, operating at 0.74 MHz, they used preacquired CT data of the skull to determine necessary corrections in the directionality of indi-vidual ultrasound elements, to accommodate aberrations in the skull surface. A stereotactic frame ensured that CT and transducer data could be coregistered. They demonstrated less than 1 mm accuracy in targeting their focal points. This algorithm introduced noninvasive transcranial FUS surgery and therapy.

MODERN FOCUSED ULTRASOUND

With Clement and Hynynen obviating craniectomy, transcranial MRgFUS research and development flourished. Thermal ablation, blood–brain barrier disruption, and neuromodulation modalities were investigated to treat movement disorders, pain, psychiatric disorders, brain neoplasms, and other diseases.[5]

The history of modern FUS is fairly recent. The most common MRgFUS systems in use today are ExAblate Neuro by Insightec, Inc, NaviFUS, and CarThera SonoCloud, with ExAblate being the most widely studied and used.[1] The ExAblate sys-tem features a hemispherical phased array of 1024 ultrasound transducers operating at 650 kHz for ablative applications and 220 kHz for blood–brain barrier opening and neuromodulation. A CT scan is performed to determine skull aberrations and density, the head is fixated in a stereotactic frame, degassed chilled water is filed between a dia-phragm around the head and the array, and the pa-tient sits awake on the MR imaging table, undergoing MR imaging and thermometry with intermittent clinical evaluations as ablative temper-atures are reached.[59]

In the recent decade, MRgFUS ablation has been used to treatment essential tremor, Parkin-son's disease, neuropathic pain, obsessive compulsive disorder, major depressive disorder, and focal hand dystonia.[3,4,60–64] Many indications are in trial phase as highlighted in other articles in this issue of MRI Clinics. MRgFUS thalamotomy and pallidotomy offer an alternative to patients who may prefer not to undergo DBS or are ineli-gible for DBS. As well, it potentially provides a one-time treatment, low maintenance alternative for the elderly.[65]

Using the low-frequency 220 kHz system, the blood–brain barrier can be reliably and reversibly opened. With the intravenous delivery of micro-bubbles, the low frequency induce their oscillation that can spatiotemporally relax endothelial–endothelial connections, allowing for both drug de-livery and for leakage of circulating tumor DNA, which can be sampled for a liquid biopsy. This method is being utilized to deliver therapeutics to treat Alzheimer's disease, high-grade gliomas, and for liquid biopsy of high-grade gliomas.[66–68] Without microbubbles, at low frequency, FUS can cause temporary alterations in neuronal activ-ity, a form of neuromodulation, which is being tri-aled for psychiatric diseases.[69]

SUMMARY

The history of transcranial FUS reveals several lessons for those interested in imaging the brain and treating neurologic and psychiatric diseases. Multidisciplinary teams consisting of physicists, engineers, neurologists, radiologists, and neuro-surgeons needed to collaborate to push the field forward. This should be encouraging to readers to continue to cross academic silos to achieve re-sults. As well, sometimes in scientific discovery, happenstance, or serendipity lends a hand, and it is difficult to predict. As Louis Pasteur said, "In the fields of observation chance favors only the prepared mind." Even as other modalities, like radiofrequency ablation, pharmacotherapy, radio-surgery, and DBS dominated the field, a few pio-neers persisted, which is motivating to all those who endeavor in the periphery. Finally, it is not lost on anyone the tremendous role that advance-ments in MR imaging have played in the develop-ment of this "noninvasive brain surgery." From the early ventriculograms chasing shadows to ablate the ansa lenticularis, to CT evaluation of the skull, to MR thermometry, to ultrasound itself, this pro-cedure owes almost everything to imaging advancement.

Today, MRgFUS faces new challenges. Patients with a low skull density ratios, the ratio of density of cancellous to cortical bone, experience difficulty in reaching ablative temperatures.[70] Because of the scattering effect of the skull, a treatment envelop exists, in which central targets are easier to lesion than peripheral targets in the brain.[71,72] The treatment still requires a full head shave. To improve clinical outcome, MR methods like trac-tography are assisting for optimal targeting.[73] The story of how the predecessors of FUS over-came their challenges serve as an inspiration to tackle these new obstacles to continue improving this technology of our future.

CLINICS CARE POINTS

- MR Guided Focused Ultrasound has evolved into a therapeutic tool with applications throughout the body
- Lack of need for brain penetration, high level of precision and real time feedback loop allow awake outpatient surgical procedures
- Existing challenges in widespread adoption relate to high cost of the systems, lack of 3D thermometry and difficulty reaching targets at the periphery of the brain for ablative purposes.

DISCLOSURE

D. Gandhi reports grants from Microvention, the Focused Ultrasound Foundation, United States, the NIH, United States and University of Calgary, United States/NoNo Therapeutics. All other authors declared no potential conflicts of interest with respect to the research, authorship, and/or publication of this article.

REFERENCES

1. Meng Y, Hynynen K, Lipsman N. Applications of focused ultrasound in the brain: from thermoablation to drug delivery. Nat Rev Neurol 2021;17(1):7–22.
2. Bond AE, Shah BB, Huss DS, et al. Safety and efficacy of focused ultrasound thalamotomy for patients with medication-refractory, tremor-dominant parkinson disease: a randomized clinical trial. JAMA Neurol 2017;74(12):1412–8.
3. Elias WJ, Lipsman N, Ondo WG, et al. A randomized trial of focused ultrasound thalamotomy for essential tremor. N Engl J Med 2016;375(8):730–9.
4. Krishna V, Fishman PS, Eisenberg HM, et al. Trial of globus pallidus focused ultrasound ablation in parkinson's disease. N Engl J Med 2023;388(8):683–93.
5. Khanna N, Gandhi D, Steven A, et al. Intracranial applications of MR imaging–guided focused ultrasound. AJNR Am J Neuroradiol 2017;38(3):426–31.
6. Curie J, Curie P. Développement par compression de l'électricité polaire dans les cristaux hémièdres à faces inclinées. Bull Mineral 1880;90–3.
7. Lippmann G. Principe de la conservation de l'électricité, ou second principe de la théorie des phénomènes électriques. J Phys Theor Appl 1881;10(1):381–94.
8. Curie J, Curie P. Contractions et dilatations produites par des tensions électriques dans les cristaux hémièdres à faces inclinées. Compt Rend 1881;93:1137–40.
9. Mason WP. Piezoelectricity, its history and applications. J Acoust Soc Am 1981;70(6):1561–6.
10. Duck F. Paul Langevin, U-boats, and ultrasonics. Phys Today 2022;75(11):42–8.
11. Kaproth-Joslin KA, Nicola R, Dogra VS. The history of us: from bats and boats to the bedside and beyond: RSNA centennial article. Radiographics 2015;35(3):960–70.
12. Dussik KT. Über die Möglichkeit, hochfrequente mechanische Schwingungen als diagnostisches Hilfsmittel zu verwerten. Arch Psychiatr Nervenkr Z Gesamte Neurol Psychiatr 1942;174(1):153–68.
13. Dussik KT. Weitere ergebnisse der ultraschalluntersuchung bei gehirnerkrankungen. Acta Neurochir (Wien) 1952;2(3):379–401.
14. Güttner W, Fiedler G, Patzold J. Über Ultraschallabbildungen am menschlichen Schädel. Acta Acust United Acust 1952;2(4):148–56.
15. Ballantine HT Jr, Hueter TF, Bolt RH. On the use of ultrasound for tumor detection. J Acoust Soc Am 1954;26(4):581.
16. Miller DL, Smith NB, Bailey MR, et al, Bioeffects Committee of the American Institute of Ultrasound in Medicine. Overview of therapeutic ultrasound applications and safety considerations. J Ultrasound Med 2012;31(4):623–34.
17. Gruetzmacher J. Piezoelektrischer Kristall mit Ultraschallkonvergenz. Zeitschrift für Physik 1935;96(5):342–9.
18. Lynn JG, Zwemer RL, Chick AJ, et al. A new method for the generation and use of focused ultrasound in experimental biology. J Gen Physiol 1942;26(2):179–93.
19. Lynn JG, Putnam TJ. Histology of cerebral lesions produced by focused ultrasound. Am J Pathol 1944;20(3):637–49.
20. O'Brien WD Jr, Dunn F. An early history of high-intensity focused ultrasound. Phys Today 2015;68(10):40–5.
21. Fry WJ. Mechanism of acoustic absorption in tissue. J Acoust Soc Am 1952;24(4):412–5.
22. Fry WJ, Fry RB. Temperature changes produced in tissue during ultrasonic irradiation. J Acoust Soc Am 1953;25(1):6–11.
23. Fry WJ, Tucker D, Fry FJ, et al. Physical factors involved in ultrasonically induced changes in living systems: II. Amplitude duration relations and the effect of hydrostatic pressure for nerve tissue. J Acoust Soc Am 1951;23(3):364–8.
24. Fry WJ, Wulff VJ, Tucker D, et al. Physical factors involved in ultrasonically induced changes in living systems: I. Identification of non-temperature effects. J Acoust Soc Am 1950;22(6):867–76.
25. Wall PD, Fry WJ, Stephens R, et al. Changes produced in the central nervous system by ultrasound. Science 1951;114(2974):686–7.

26. Fry WJ, Fry FJ, Barnard JW, et al. Ultrasonic lesions in the mammalian central nervous system. Science 1955;122(3168):517–8.

27. Fry WJ, Mosberg WH, Barnard JW, et al. Production of focal destructive lesions in the central nervous system with ultrasound. J Neurosurg 1954;11(5): 471–8.

28. Rahman M, Murad GJ, Mocco J. Early history of the stereotactic apparatus in neurosurgery. Neurosurg Focus 2009;27(3):E12.

29. Abel TJ, Walch T, Howard MA 3rd. Russell Meyers (1905-1999): pioneer of functional and ultrasonic neurosurgery. J Neurosurg 2016;125(6): 1589–95.

30. Benabid AL, Chabardes S, Torres N, et al. Functional neurosurgery for movement disorders: a historical perspective. Prog Brain Res 2009;175:379–91.

31. Gabriel EM, Nashold BS Jr. Evolution of neuroablative surgery for involuntary movement disorders: an historical review. Neurosurgery 1998;42(3):575–90. discussion 590-571.

32. Guridi J, Lozano AM. A brief history of pallidotomy. Neurosurgery 1997;41(5):1169–80. discussion 1180-1163.

33. Meyers R. The extrapyramidal system. Neurology 1953;3(9):627.

34. Dandy W. Changes in our conceptions oj localization of certain functions in the brain. American Journal of Physiology 1930;93:643.

35. Meyers R. Surgical experiments in the therapy of certain 'extrapyramidal' diseases: a current evaluation. Acta psychiatrica et neurologica. Supplementum 1951;67:1–42.

36. Meyers R, Fry WJ, Fry FJ, et al. Early experiences with ultrasonic irradiation of the pallidofugal and nigral complexes in hyperkinetic and hypertonic disorders. J Neurosurg 1959;16(1):32–54.

37. Editors. Ultrasound Surgery. Time Magazine 1957 (Dec 02): 37.

38. Fry WJ, Fry FJ. Fundamental neurological research and human neurosurgery using intense ultrasound. IRE Trans Biomed Electron 1960;Me-7:166–81.

39. Spiegel EA, Wycis HT, Marks M, et al. Stereotaxic apparatus for operations on the human brain. Science 1947;106(2754):349–50.

40. Cooper IS, Bravo G. Chemopallidectomy and chemothalamectomy. J Neurosurg 1958;15(3):244–50.

41. Svennilson E, Torvik A, Lowe R, et al. Treatment of parkinsonism by stereotatic thermolesions in the pallidal region. A clinical evaluation of 81 cases. Acta Psychiatr Scand 1960;35(3):358–77.

42. Leksell L. Cerebral radiosurgery. I. Gammathalanotomy in two cases of intractable pain. Acta Chir Scand 1968;134(8):585–95.

43. Frighetto L, Bizzi J, Annes RD, et al. Stereotactic radiosurgery for movement disorders. Surg Neurol Int 2012;3(Suppl 1):S10–6.

44. Carlsson A, Lindqvist M, Magnusson TOR. 3,4-dihydroxyphenylalanine and 5-hydroxytryptophan as reserpine antagonists. Nature 1957;180(4596):1200.

45. Cotzias GC, Van Woert MH, Schiffer LM. Aromatic amino acids and modification of parkinsonism. N Engl J Med 1967;276(7):374–9.

46. Ehringer H, Hornykiewicz O. [Distribution of noradrenaline and dopamine (3-hydroxytyramine) in the human brain and their behavior in diseases of the extrapyramidal system]. Klinische Wochenschrift 1960;38:1236–9.

47. Benabid AL, Pollak P, Louveau A, et al. Combined (thalamotomy and stimulation) stereotactic surgery of the VIM thalamic nucleus for bilateral Parkinson disease. Appl Neurophysiol 1987;50(1–6): 344–6.

48. Krauss JK, Lipsman N, Aziz T, et al. Technology of deep brain stimulation: current status and future directions. Nat Rev Neurol 2021;17(2):75–87.

49. Heimburger RF, Eggleton RC, Fry FJ. Ultrasonic visualization in determination of tumor growth rate. JAMA 1973;224(4):497–501.

50. Heimburger RF, Fry FJ, Eggleton RC. Ultrasound visualization in human brain: the internal capsule, a preliminary report. Surg Neurol 1973;1(1):56–8.

51. Heimburger RF, Fry FJ, Franklin TD, et al. Ultrasound diagnosis for head injuries. J Indiana State Med Assoc 1976;69(5):247–50.

52. Heimburger RF, Fry FJ, Franklin TD, et al. Two dimensional ultrasound scanning of excised brains-I. Normal anatomy. Ultrasound Med Biol 1977;2(4): 279–85.

53. Heimburger RF. Ultrasound augmentation of central nervous system tumor therapy. J Indiana State Med Assoc 1985;78(6):469–76.

54. Guthkelch AN, Carter LP, Cassady JR, et al. Treatment of malignant brain tumors with focused ultrasound hyperthermia and radiation: results of a phase I trial. J Neurooncol 1991;10(3):271–84.

55. Hynynen K, Damianou C, Darkazanli A, et al. The feasibility of using MRI to monitor and guide noninvasive ultrasound surgery. Ultrasound Med Biol 1993;19(1):91–2.

56. Hynynen K, Jolesz FA. Demonstration of potential noninvasive ultrasound brain therapy through an intact skull. Ultrasound Med Biol 1998;24(2): 275–83.

57. Vimeux FC, De Zwart JA, Palussiére J, et al. Real-time control of focused ultrasound heating based on rapid MR thermometry. Invest Radiol 1999;34(3):190–3.

58. Clement GT, Hynynen K. A non-invasive method for focusing ultrasound through the human skull. Phys Med Biol 2002;47(8):1219–36.

59. Jameel A, Bain P, Nandi D, et al. Device profile of exAblate Neuro 4000, the leading system for brain magnetic resonance guided focused ultrasound technology: an overview of its safety and efficacy

in the treatment of medically refractory essential tremor. Expert Rev Med Devices 2021;18(5):429–37.

60. Ahmed A-K, Zhuo J, Gullapalli RP, et al. Focused ultrasound central lateral thalamotomy for the treatment of refractory neuropathic pain: phase I trial. Neurosurgery 2024;94(4):690–9.

61. Ishaque M, Moosa S, Urban L, et al. Bilateral focused ultrasound medial thalamotomies for trigeminal neuropathic pain: a randomized controlled study. J Neurosurg 2023;1–11.

62. Jeanmonod D, Werner B, Morel A, et al. Transcranial magnetic resonance imaging-guided focused ultrasound: noninvasive central lateral thalamotomy for chronic neuropathic pain. Neurosug Focus 2012; 32(1):E1.

63. Davidson B, Hamani C, Meng Y, et al. Examining cognitive change in magnetic resonance-guided focused ultrasound capsulotomy for psychiatric illness. Transl Psychiatry 2020;10(1):397.

64. Horisawa S, Yamaguchi T, Abe K, et al. Magnetic resonance-guided focused ultrasound thalamotomy for focal hand dystonia: a pilot Study. Mov Disord 2021;36(8):1955–9.

65. Paff M, Boutet A, Neudorfer C, et al. Magnetic resonance-guided focused ultrasound thalamotomy to treat essential tremor in nonagenarians. Stereotact Funct Neurosurg 2020;98(3):182–6.

66. Anastasiadis P, Gandhi D, Guo Y, et al. Localized blood–brain barrier opening in infiltrating gliomas with MRI-guided acoustic emissions–controlled focused ultrasound. Proc Natl Acad Sci U S A 2021;118(37). e2103280118.

67. Meng Y, Pople CB, Suppiah S, et al. MR-guided focused ultrasound liquid biopsy enriches circulating biomarkers in patients with brain tumors. Neuro Oncol 2021;23(10):1789–97.

68. Rezai AR, D'Haese P-F, Finomore V, et al. Ultrasound blood–brain barrier opening and aducanumab in Alzheimer's disease. N Engl J Med 2024;390(1):55–62.

69. Arulpragasam AR, van 't Wout-Frank M, Barredo J, et al. Low intensity focused ultrasound for noninvasive and reversible deep brain neuromodulation-a paradigm shift in psychiatric research. Front Psychiatry 2022;13:825802.

70. D'Souza M, Chen KS, Rosenberg J, et al. Impact of skull density ratio on efficacy and safety of magnetic resonance–guided focused ultrasound treatment of essential tremor. J Neurosurg 2020 2020;132(5): 1392–7.

71. Meng Y, Jones RM, Davidson B, et al. Technical principles and clinical workflow of transcranial mr-guided focused ultrasound. Stereotact Funct Neurosurg 2020;99(4):329–42.

72. Ahmed AK, Guo S, Kelm N, et al. Technical comparison of treatment efficiency of magnetic resonance-guided focused ultrasound thalamotomy and pallidotomy in skull density ratio-matched patient cohorts. Front Neurology 2021; 12:808810.

73. Feltrin FS, Chopra R, Pouratian N, et al. Focused ultrasound using a novel targeting method four-tract tractography for magnetic resonance-guided high-intensity focused ultrasound targeting. Brain Commun 2022;4(6):fcac273.

MR Imaging-Guided Focused Ultrasound for Breast Tumors

Matthew DeWitt, PhD[a,b], Zehra E.F. Demir, BS[a], Thomas Sherlock, BS[a],
David R. Brenin, MD[b,c], Natasha D. Sheybani, PhD[a,b,d],*

KEYWORDS

- MR imaging • Focused ultrasound • Breast tumors • Cancer • Fibroadenoma • Metastasis
- Ablation

KEY POINTS

- Given the invasive nature of traditional surgery, there remains a critical need for improved breast tumor interventions across both benign and malignant settings.
- MR imaging-guided focused ultrasound (FUS) technology offers a promising noninvasive, non-ionizing approach for spatially precise thermal ablation of breast tumors in the primary setting.
- Additional strategies showcase the versatility of MR imaging-guided FUS for intervention at distal breast cancer sites, with applications advancing for thermal ablation for pain palliation of bone metastases or blood–brain barrier opening in brain metastases.

INTRODUCTION

Breast tumors, both benign and malignant, persist as a widespread and intricate health challenge on a global scale. In particular, breast cancer is now the most frequently diagnosed and second leading cause of cancer-related deaths in women, affirming its significance as a global health burden.[1] In 2023, there were an estimated over 300,000 new breast cancer cases diagnosed in the United States. There were over 43,000 deaths due to breast cancer over that same time period. Breast cancer mortalities are attributable to metastatic spread to distal sites such as lungs, liver, bone, and brain at later stages of disease.[2] Indeed, whereas localized breast cancers have a 5 year survival rate of 99%, this survival rate is markedly lower in patients who have metastatic (stage IV) disease (31%).[3] To date, metastatic breast cancer remains incurable, with limited treatment options available.[4] Increased screening and improved imaging technologies have led to earlier detection of breast cancer, which aids in reducing the mortality associated with later stage and metastatic disease.[5] However, the increased surveillance has also resulted in increased detection of benign lesions such as fibroadenomas (FAs), which can vary radically in size, occasionally growing large enough to cause significant discomfort or cosmetic concern.

Surgical resection (ie, lumpectomy or mastectomy), albeit highly invasive, has traditionally been a mainstay for both benign and malignant primary breast tumor removal. While effective, this approach harbors significant physical and psychological impacts for patients, including prolonged recovery times, scarring, and disfigurement. In settings of malignancy, surgical resection is often

[a] Department of Biomedical Engineering, University of Virginia, Charlottesville, VA, USA; [b] Focused Ultrasound Cancer Immunotherapy Center, University of Virginia, Charlottesville, VA, USA; [c] Division of Surgical Oncology, University of Virginia Health System, Charlottesville, VA, USA; [d] Department of Radiology & Medical Imaging, University of Virginia, Charlottesville, VA, USA
* Corresponding author. Department of Biomedical Engineering, Health System, University of Virginia, Box 800759, Charlottesville, VA 22908.
E-mail address: nds3sa@virginia.edu

Magn Reson Imaging Clin N Am 32 (2024) 593–613
https://doi.org/10.1016/j.mric.2024.04.004

accompanied by radiation therapy and chemotherapy, which contribute additional off-target toxicities that can be debilitating for patients. Encouragingly, the past 2 decades have seen a dramatic shift toward de-escalation of surgeries and emphasis on tumor biology—catalyzing the advent of breast-conserving treatments. This move toward tissue-sparing approaches is especially promising in the management of benign lesions, where more conservative monitoring is typically employed until lesions become painful and require treatment. The paradigm shift away from traditional surgical interventions toward less invasive, less toxic alternatives is driven by the evolving understanding of the disease and patient-centered care approaches and can lead to a cosmetically superior outcome and reduce the psychological burden associated with surgical procedures.

Minimally invasive treatment options, such as ablation (eg, focused ultrasound [FUS] ablation, microwave thermotherapy, radiofrequency ablation, laser ablation, and cryoablation), radiotherapy, and targeted drug therapies, offer marked potential in the advancement of breast cancer therapy.[6] These options may be particularly beneficial for patients with comorbidities, who might be at higher risk for surgical complications and the ability to perform these treatments in an outpatient setting can potentially lower the health care costs and resource utilization associated with traditional surgical management of breast cancer and FAs. Moreover, the shift toward these techniques aligns with a broader trend in medicine toward personalized care, aiming not only to treat the disease effectively but also to enhance the overall well-being and lifestyle of patients during and after treatment. This patient-centric approach is particularly crucial in breast cancer, where the implications of treatment can extend far beyond physical health, impacting psychological and social aspects of life.

Among the aforementioned interventions, only FUS is truly noninvasive, resulting in the potential for reduced pain, lower risk of infection, and minimal scaring associated with invasive or minimally invasive technologies. The nonionizing energy enables repeat treatments which can be important in cases where lesions may recur, or new ones develop. Additionally, FUS has a unique versatility to enable bioeffects beyond ablation, accompanied by unique capabilities for treatment planning, guidance, and control. FUS has evolved from a relatively unexplored research tool for noninvasive tissue destruction, which was only employed at select academic clinical locations with custom devices, to a meaningful treatment option with

equipment developed by numerous manufacturers and under investigation worldwide for the treatment of breast tumors. This review highlights the clinical advancement of FUS technology—with an emphasis on MR imaging-guided FUS—for benign FAs and breast cancers spanning the primary and metastatic settings.

OVERVIEW OF FOCUSED ULTRASOUND TECHNOLOGY

Therapeutic FUS is typically delivered either by a single or multiple, precisely aligned concave piezoelectric transducers which can generate an energy density of approximately 10 W/cm^2 at the surface of the transducer and, due to the focusing of the ultrasound beam, can reach intensities greater than 2000 W/cm^2 at the focal point. The concave shape of the transducer ensures that waves converge to a predictable single point. This focal spot is typically cylindrical or ellipsoidal in shape, and the size can range from 5 to 60 mm in length and 2 to 15 mm in diameter. While diagnostic or imaging ultrasound transducers typically operate in the 2 to 15 MHz range, therapeutic FUS devices typically employ frequencies ranging from hundreds of kilohertz to 3 MHz.

When FUS energy is delivered, the tissue absorption in the focal spot and along the beam path is critical for establishing the resulting bioeffect.[7] If the ultrasound energy is delivered as a continuous waveform, the absorption of energy within the focal spot can raise the temperature significantly within a few seconds. The noninvasive and spatially precise targeting enabled by FUS technology are owing to acoustic parameters—and, in some cases, beam steering capabilities—that can be tuned to drive significant energy deposition in the focal spot while minimizing effects along the intervening beam path, including the skin and nontarget tissue. Thermal effects can range from hyperthermia (40–45°C),[8] where the sublethal elevation in temperature has been leveraged for therapeutic delivery and radiosensitization or higher temperatures (>55°C) for thermal coagulation. Numerous clinical studies have demonstrated that thermal FUS is a sensitizer of radiotherapy in different cancers, including those of the head and neck, breast, and prostate.[9] FUS can also be delivered using high instantaneous powers and low duty cycles, such that the pressure at the focus is greater than the intrinsic limit of the tissue, resulting in primarily mechanical effects without significant heating, that is, histotripsy.[10] While not yet widely accessible for the clinical treatment of breast cancer, there is growing evidence for the use of histotripsy for soft tissue ablation and hepatocellular carcinoma.[11,12] Numerous preclinical studies support the implementation of this technology across tumor debulking and immunotherapy applications,[13] among others, in the breast.[14] Additionally, low-power and low duty cycle pulses can be coupled with systemically delivered microbubbles to drive dramatic shifts in localized pressure within blood vessels in the focal region, an approach which can be useful for transiently perturbing the vasculature for improved local drug delivery.[15]

The majority of clinical applications for FUS in breast cancer—including primary breast cancer, benign lesions (ie, FAs), and metastatic lesions—exploit high-intensity FUS (HIFU) for thermal ablation.[16] HIFU devices aim to thermally destroy deleterious tissues by subjecting tissue at the focus to temperature exceeding 56°C, where nearly instantaneous (>1 second) exposure results in focal tissue coagulation, protein denaturation, and a transitional margin of cell damage and death (termed the periablative zone).[17] Larger ablation lesions are generated by steering the transducers to multiple focal spots. More recent approaches utilize lower applied powers to induce hyperthermia to enhance chemotherapy delivery from thermosensitive drug-bearing liposomes such as ThermoDox[18] which are initiating clinical translation for breast cancer treatment.[19] Overall, the noninvasive nature of FUS, irrespective of modality, enables reduced side effects compared to invasive surgical interventions, and the nonionizing applied energy readily enables repeat interventions where necessary. An overview of the most advanced therapeutic mechanism of action for FUS across primary, benign, and metastatic breast tumor contexts is provided in **Fig. 1**.

FUS devices used to treat breast masses can generally be classified into 2 categories: ultrasound-guided FUS (USgFUS; **Fig. 2**) or MR imaging-guided FUS (MRgFUS; **Fig. 3**), based on the imaging modality utilized during treatment. The use of USgFUS is generally considered more economical due to lower FUS and image guiding instrumentation costs and reduced setup times.[16,20] However, MRgFUS enables higher resolution treatment planning and the potential for real-time temperature feedback which can improve safety, efficiency, and precision.[21]

There are two main device designs encompassed within the MRgFUS category. The first uses a vertical ultrasound beam with a single transducer integrated into the MR imaging tabletop. A dedicated FUS workstation enables image fusion and treatment planning, along with transducer control and temperature monitoring capabilities. Initially, custom systems of this design were used

in early trials based in Germany.[22] In more recent years, a commercially available clinical MRgFUS system was developed by Insightec Ltd—the Ex-Ablate 2000 (InSightec, Israel). This commercial device has been advanced for thermally ablative interventions in the uterus, breast, prostate, brain, and bone.[23] In this approach, the patient's breast is positioned in the center of the MR surface coil and are both lowered into an MR imaging platform that contains the 1.15 MHz therapeutic ultrasound transducer.[24] The platform is filled with degassed water to ensure proper acoustic coupling to the transducer. During the procedure, the degassed water is circulated and maintained at 20°C to provide active cooling of the skin. Temperature is mapped using the proton resonance frequency (PRF) shift methods and is used to ensure complete heating without off-target effects. A second, more recent, approach for MRgFUS procedures is offered by the Sonalleve System (Profound Medical, Canada).[25] This device uses eight 1.2 MHz transducer modules in a breast-specific cup that treats lesions laterally, such that the far-field energy remains in the breast tissue.[26] The device employs a double-membrane system with cooled water for coupling and reduced surface heating. Recent advances in the geometry of the array of transducers may enable improved thermal volumes in heterogenous tissues while additionally allowing higher pressures to be applied for next-generation histotripsy applications.[27]

Both MRgFUS systems offer real-time thermometry, enabling adjustment of the treatment plan and ultrasound settings to ensure complete volumetric heating of the targeted lesion with high anatomic resolution and sensitivity to thermal rise within the focal volume.[28] Despite these significant advantages, the major drawback of MRgFUS in this context is the high cost, the need for additional support staffing, and the extended setup time resulting in long procedural times (>1 hour) despite the usually fast ablation times (<20 minutes). Additionally, the proton phase shift-based measurements used for temperature mapping can be unreliable due to the high amount of fat in the breast.

USgFUS employs conventional diagnostic ultrasound imaging for treatment guidance; in contrast with MRgFUS, USgFUS does not readily enable thermography to monitor and adapt treatment. As such, most clinical studies of USgFUS, thermal ablation zone temperatures have not been directly measured.[29] Instead, changes in echogenicity in B-mode imaging are used as feedback for the level of coagulative necrosis present. USgFUS requires the tumor to be visible on ultrasound and for the lesion to be at least 5 mm from the skin or chest

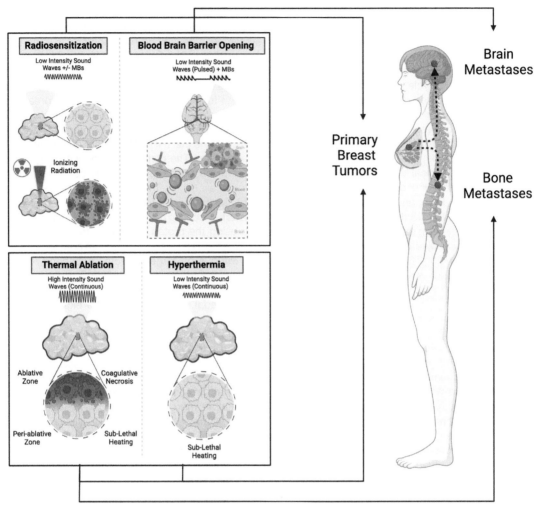

Fig. 1. Focused ultrasound strategies under clinical investigation for treatment of breast tumors. (Created with Biorender.com.)

wall. The two primary USgFUS devices that have been utilized in breast lesioning trials include the Model-JC HIFU system (Haifu Technology, Chongqing, China) and the Echopulse (Theraclion, Malakoff, France). The Model-JC HIFU system utilizes a tabletop approach that integrates a 3.5 MHz imaging transducer with a 1.6 MHz therapeutic transducer. The target lesion is identified with B-mode imaging and the therapeutic probe is translated until the predicted focal spot overlaps the lesion. The Echopulse device utilizes a 3.0 MHz therapeutic transducer mounted on a rotatable arm for proper positioning and delivery of energy. An integrated 7.5 to 12 MHz imaging transducer, colocalized with the HIFU transducer, is used for lesion identification and treatment visualization.

We provide an overview of key studies and clinical findings that demonstrate the great promise of these two classes of devices in the noninvasive treatment of primary, benign, and metastatic breast tumors.

APPLICATIONS OF IMAGE-GUIDED FOCUSED ULTRASOUND IN BREAST TUMORS
Primary Breast Cancers

The first reports of FUS for the ablation of primary breast cancer were disseminated from China as a part of broader investigations using USgFUS for ablation of mixed soft tissue malignancies.[30] This study established safety and offered early evidence of efficacy by MR imaging follow-up in over 100 patients. Huber and colleagues[22] performed the first investigation of MRgFUS thermal ablation for core biopsy-proven breast cancer using a custom 1.7 MHz system and followed with

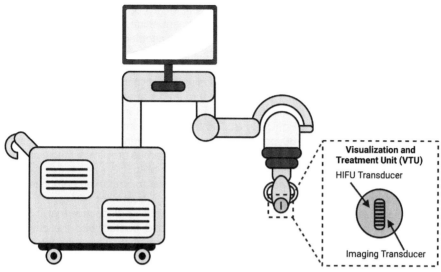

Fig. 2. Ultrasound-guided focused ultrasound. Representative schematic depicting adjustable ultrasound-guided FUS device (eg, theraclion echopulse system) comprised of therapeutic ultrasound transducer with embedded ultrasound imaging array. VTU, visualization and treatment unit. (Created with Biorender.com.)

histopathological analysis of the resected tumor following breast conserving surgery. This study demonstrated successful ablation of the targeted tumor in a single patient without damage to proximal healthy tissue or skin. Since the establishment of initial feasibility, the major goals of clinical MRgFUS investigations in breast cancer have been to define the appropriate patient population including stage and tumor size, demonstrate successful feedback-monitored energy deposition yielding tumor necrosis, decrease total procedural time, and fortify evidence for positive patient response.

Following the commercial development of the Exablate 2000 system, larger clinical trials were initiated in Japan, Israel, and Canada to evaluate safety, feasibility, and efficacy of MRgFUS in infiltrating breast cancer. Gianfelice and colleagues[31,32] evaluated MRgFUS with the Exablate system in approximately 30 patients with a mean breast cancer diameter of 1.5 cm. In the first 12 patient cohort, resection was performed immediately following treatment; meanwhile, a second 17 patient study employed follow-up radiologic evaluation and resection within 21 days of treatment. Despite demonstrating safety, only 43% of cancer tissue was identified as sufficiently necrosed, with only 17% of patients exhibiting complete necrosis. After the Exablate system was upgraded to the Mark2 system, which enhanced

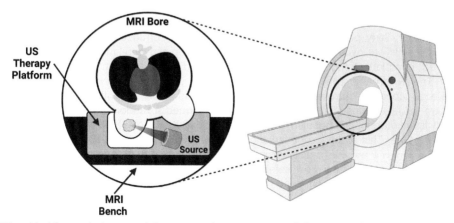

Fig. 3. MRI-guided focused ultrasound. Representative cross-sectional depiction of an MR imaging-guided FUS device framework for treatment of primary breast tumors. (Created with Biorender.com.)

the targeting protocol, they demonstrated 89% complete cancer necrosis. Additional studies with longer follow-up performed by this group showed no viable tumor in 59% of patients treated with FUS in an adjuvant setting alongside systemic tamoxifen.[32]

Among their numerous published studies assessing MRgFUS for breast tumor ablation, Furusawa and colleagues[33] evaluated MRgFUS in a prospective treat-and-resect trial of 30 patients with unknown stages of breast cancer, with lesions less than 3.5 cm in diameter. Their findings from histologic analysis of resected specimens taken 2 weeks post-treatment demonstrated a mean of 97% tumor ablation volume, with 60% of cases reflecting complete tumor ablation and a single case demonstrating less than 95% tumor ablation.[34] Only one adverse event (skin burn) was noted and 2 patients reported mild pain during treatment, fortifying the feasibility of safe lesioning procedures without major complications. Cavallo Marincola, and colleagues evaluated MRgFUS in 10 patients in a nonrandomized treat-and-resect study in invasive ductal carcinoma patients with an average tumor diameter of 1.2 cm.[35] Treatment time averaged 140 minutes. While no adverse events were noted, 20% of patients demonstrated residual tumor enhancement in MR imaging evaluation post-treatment and an additional 20% of patients showed histopathological evidence of viable tumor cells in the ablative zone, signifying a 60% overall success rate. No evidence of recurrence was seen in any patients following resection. Taken together, these studies demonstrated early success of MRgFUS for the treatment of breast cancer and reflected opportunities for improvement in complete ablation efficacy and minimization of total treatment time.

Recent studies utilizing the MRgFUS Sonalleve system have demonstrated significantly faster treatment times, with an average procedure time of 57 minutes and with no patients exhibiting skin redness or burns.[36] Sixty percent of the 10 patients enrolled in a clinical investigation of the system displayed complete tumor necrosis after treatment.[37] Toward broader clinical adoption, it is imperative to conduct comprehensive trials with long-term follow-up, ensuring that the treatment not only is effective initially but also prevents recurrence over time. This extended observation and data collection will provide crucial insights regarding the long-term efficacy and safety of FUS ablation, thereby bolstering confidence in its use as a reliable and complete treatment modality. Ongoing trials with the Sonalleve device (BRIFU trial; NCT02407613) will expand this knowledge gap, with resection occurring 30 days following treatment to broaden the window for assessing treatment efficacy.

In yet another recent advancement, a first-in-human trial is now investigating a custom breast-specific Muse MRgFUS system developed at the University of Utah (NCT05291507). This system integrates an advanced targeting mechanism and volumetric MR imaging protocols for more accurate in-treatment temperature and lesion monitoring. Clinical investigation of this system builds upon numerous preclinical studies aimed at developing the MRgFUS system that can address the critical need for improved complete ablation while minimizing treatment times.[38,39] In an early readout of this prospective trial, 10 patients were enrolled and treated with the custom system.[40] Average treatment time was 92 minutes (range: 73–114 minutes), and importantly, no adverse events were noted. The use of a 3D MR thermometry approach in this study also offers potential for overcoming "undertreatment" observed in earlier trials utilizing PRF imaging for temperature monitoring—specifically by providing enhanced real-time feedback inclusive of changes in adipose tissue, which was a limitation of PRF methods employed in early MRgFUS investigations.[41] This complete trial will enroll up to 34 patients with tumor resection up to 6 weeks following ablation.

In tandem with investigations of MRgFUS, applications of USgFUS in breast tumors have burgeoned as well. USgFUS has predominantly been evaluated in China for primary breast cancer ablation, with multiple reports having been published on early experiences by Wu and colleagues.[42] Initial trials demonstrated the safety of USgFUS in 23 patients with breast cancer having undergone a treat-and-resect protocol within a 2 week time frame.[43] In these studies, complete ablation was noted in 100% of patients, with an average treatment time of 78 minutes, and only a single adverse event composed of a minor skin burn. Follow-on studies from Wu and colleagues[44] showed recurrence in 2 of 22 patients with a mean follow-up of over 54 months. Kim and colleagues[45] treated 6 patients and performed MR imaging follow-up, demonstrating complete ablation in 4 patients. More recently, Guan and colleagues[46] performed a randomized controlled trial with the Model-JC USgFUS device and demonstrated complete ablation in 100% of patients with an average treatment time of 66 minutes and 5 year disease-free survival of 95%.

As is the case with MRgFUS, the efficacy of treatment with USgFUS is highly dependent on accurate real-time treatment monitoring. Presently, commercially available USgFUS devices employ B-mode imaging feedback for treatment planning and guidance. On occasion, hyperechoic marks appear on imaging following ablation, reflective of boiling activity at elevated temperatures. Alternative to B-mode imaging, wherein such signatures offer a purely qualitative form of feedback, the advent of harmonic motion imaging (HMI) offers promise of improved feedback.[47] HMI is an acoustic radiation force-based elasticity imaging technique that can offer improved contrast resolution and quantitative assessment of tissue viscoelastic property changes following ablation.[48] Preclinical evidence suggests that HMI can provide more appropriate feedback than B-mode imaging for monitoring ablation progress.[49] An ongoing clinical trial at Columbia University (NCT05219695) is testing a custom HMI-guided FUS system to evaluate the efficacy of this approach in 34 patients with nonmetastatic breast cancer or FAs. Improved treatment monitoring could help overcome the main shortcoming of USgFUS and promote its use over MRgFUS, which currently provides higher resolution planning and treatment tracking.

Table 1 summarizes the clinical trials involving MRgFUS and USgFUS for primary breast cancer ablation. Studies completed in this space to date have demonstrated the promise of FUS for primary breast cancer ablation, while highlighting opportunities for technological improvements in treatment planning and real-time feedback approaches to ensure margin status, as well as continued measures to ensure cost-effectiveness of the procedure (eg, through reduced treatment times). As will be discussed further, recent or ongoing studies are also investigating FUS thermal ablation of breast cancers in combination with systemic chemotherapy (NCT04796220) or immunotherapy (NCT03237572).

Breast Fibroadenomas

In addition to the use of FUS for primary breast malignancies, there is growing promise in the employment of this noninvasive technology for ablation of benign breast lesions such as FAs.[50] FAs represent the most common benign breast lesion and account for 30% to 75% of all biopsied breast lumps in young women. FAs are solid, nontender benign breast lesions commonly discovered in women between the age of 15 and 35 years. These lesions can become bothersome and can require intervention after the typical observation period of 6 to 12 months.[51]

Owing to their benign nature, conservative management with follow-up has remained the standard of care for FAs.[52] Surgical resection is an option for patients with bothersome FAs.[53] FUS ablation represents an attractive noninvasive alternative to surgery for all patients with FA, obviating the risk of surgery-related complications and the need for general anesthesia.

Much like the treatment of primary breast cancer, FUS ablation of FAs consists of pretreatment scans for treatment planning, followed by delivery of ablative energy under either MR or US guidance. Various energy levels (10–200 W) have been employed for thermal ablation of FAs depending on size, consistency, and location. Additionally, distinct treatment protocols have been deployed in FAs, including (1) complete lesion ablation with overlapping sonication spots or (2) circumferential lesioning (center of lesion deselected and only outer region of lesion targeted). A drawback of the former is the prolonged treatment time, which can take up to 3 hours to complete. Circumferential lesioning can reduce this time by nearly 40% with minimal impact to ablation success.

FUS is particularly well-suited for noninvasive debulking of FAs due to their proximity to the skin. Numerous clinical trials over the past 2 decades have been performed to evaluate the safety, feasibility, and efficacy of FUS ablation for treatment of FAs—assessing changes in FA volume and symptom improvement, noting complications or adverse events, and evaluating quality of life for up to 2 years following treatment. Across published studies to date, the success rate of FUS ablation for FA has been markedly high. Recently, Kwong and colleagues[54] reported significant reduction in FA volume following USgFUS, with follow-up over a year following treatment. Meanwhile, Kovatcheva and colleagues[55] and Peek and colleagues[56] have demonstrated significant volumetric reduction at 12 months post-FUS, with a combined mean volumetric reduction of 72% between the studies. Imankulov and colleagues[57] demonstrated higher quality of life in patients with FA treated with FUS ablation relative to those compared who underwent surgical resection, reporting 52% reduction in hospitalization duration compared to surgery and 67% higher pain scores in control (observational) patients with FA compared to FUS recipients. Hahn and colleagues[58] found that 89% of patients were satisfied with symptom diminution and 96% of would recommend the procedure to future patients. An overview of the clinical evidence for FUS ablation in the management of FAs is presented in Table 2.

Overall, FUS in the treatment of FA has been demonstrated safe and well tolerated.[59] Less than 5% of patients with FA treated with FUS suffered superficial skin burns and less than 10%

Table 1
Summary of clinical investigations of focused ultrasound in primary breast cancer

Study Identifier	Device	Cases	Stages/ Tumor Type	Size	Ablation Success	Time	Evaluation Method	Primary Outcomes
Gianfelice et al,[31] 2003; Gianfelice et al,[32] 2003*,**	Exablate 2000 MRgFUS	12, 17	Invasive breast cancer	<3.5 cm (0.1–8.8 cm³)	79% MR imaging/ 24% H&E	80 m (35–133)	MR imaging*/ histopathological**	Mean necrosis of first 3 patients of 43.3% followed by 88.3% in next 9 patients in first study. 100% necrosis in 5 patients in second study, 9 with 90% necrosis, and 4 patients with <70% necrosis. 8 moderate pain and 4 patients with slight pain. 2 cases of second-degree skin burn.
Furusawa et al,[33] 2006, Furusawa et al,[34] 2007	Exablate 2000 MRgFUS	30	Invasive breast cancer	1.3 cm	95% MR imaging/ 54% H&E	140 m (76–231)	H&E 5–23 d post-treatment	Mean necrosis of 97%. 53.4% of patients had 100% necrosis and only 3 patients had <95% necrosis. 1 patient third-degree skin burn and 5 minor adverse events. Reaffirmed the need for contrast-enhanced images for precise treatment
Zippel et al,[76] 2005	Exablate 2000 MRgFUS	10	Invasive breast cancer	2.2 cm	20%	120 m (<240 m)	H&E 7–10 d post-treatment	All patients underwent standard surgery 10 d after ablation. Only 2 of 10 patients had complete treatment and 3 of 10 had more than 10% of viable tumor remaining.

Study	Device	No.	Tumor Type	Size	%	Time	Confirmation	Outcome
Khiat et al,[77] 2006	Exablate 2000 MRgFUS	26	Invasive ductal carcinoma	3.3 cm	31%	N/A	MR imaging (dynamic contrast-enhanced) + H&E	MR imaging evaluation for 14 d prior to resection. Among the 26 treated tumors, 7 tumors showed no detectable residual cancer at the site of MRgFUS, 11 tumors had residual cancer below 10%, and 7 tumors showed a larger percentage of residual cancer, which ranged between 20% and 90%.
Cavallo Marincola et al,[35] 2015	Exablate 2000 MRgFUS	10	Invasive ductal carcinoma	1.2 cm	60%	140 m (80–180)	MR imaging + H&E within 14 d	In 6 of 10 patients, no enhancement was seen on DCE-MR imaging. In 2 of 10 patients, residual enhancing tissue was seen in MR imaging and confirmed with H&E.
Merckel et al,[36] 2013, Merckel et al,[37] 2016	Sonalleve MRgFUS	10	Invasive ductal and lobular carcinoma	2.0 cm	60%	46 m (12–75)	H&E within 2–10 d	An overall 145 min procedure time and no skin burns were observed. Two patients reported pain and 2 patients developed white bumps. Average ablation temperature was 51.4 C. Partial ablation was applied so complete ablation was not evaluated.

(continued on next page)

Table 1
(continued)

Study Identifier	Device	Cases	Stages/Tumor Type	Size	Ablation Success	Time	Evaluation Method	Primary Outcomes
Payne et al,[40] 2020	MUSE MRgFUS	10	T0-stage breast cancer	4.48 cm³	80%	92 m (73–115)	Magnetic resonance thermal MRTI	Treatments were monitored with volumetric MR-acoustic radiation force imaging and temperature mapping. Successful ablation was achieved in 80% of patients. Mean error of targeting was 6.2 mm in patients. MR-TI and -ARFI were successful in 60% and 70% of patients, respectively.
Wu et al	Model-JC HAIFU USgFUS	23	Invasive breast cancer	3.1 cm	100%	78 m (45–150)	Resection 1–2 wk	Heat fixation in the complete tumor was confirmed in all patients and USgHIFU was confirmed safe and effective with 91.3% complete necrosis identified histologically.
Wu et al	Model-JC HAIFU USgFUS	22	Invasive breast cancer	3.4 cm	100%	132 m (60–180)	Core biopsy + H&E	Complete necrosis was seen in 100% of patients. The 5 y disease-free and recurrence-free survival were 95% and 89%, respectively.

Kim et al,[45] 2010	Model-JC HAIFU USgFUS	6	Invasive ductal carcinoma	2.6 cm	67%	174 m (80–285)	Biopsy and 30 mo MR imaging follow-up	No viable tumor in 4 of the 6 treated patients with various follow-up times. Demonstrated that dynamic MR imaging following treatment provides critical information for treatment assessment.
Guan et al,[46] 2016	Model-JC HAIFU USgFUS	25	Invasive breast cancer: Stages I, IIa, and IIb	2.1–4.8 cm	100%	66 m (40–132)	Resection 1–2 wk/H&E	Coagulative necrosis was seen in 100% of patients with an included margin of 1.92 cm. No severe adverse events. 44% exhibited pain or discomfort. No vascular damage noted.
NCT05291507 (BreastMRgFUS)	MUSE MRgFUS	34	Unifocal invasive breast cancer	TBD	TBD	TBD	Resection within 6 wk	Tumors will be treated with partial ablation (50%) and resected within 6 wk of treatment for histologic analysis, imaging correlation, and safety and efficacy of the MUSE MRgFUS system.
NCT04796220 (Breast54)	Echopulse USgFUS	48	Invasive breast cancer: Stages 1–3	TBD	TBD	TBD	Resection after 22 d	Evaluate the combination of FUS thermal ablation with gemcitabine to determine efficacy and immunologic reaction in early-stage breast cancer and assess patient satisfaction.

(continued on next page)

Table 1
(continued)

Study Identifier	Device	Cases	Stages/ Tumor Type	Size	Ablation Success	Time	Evaluation Method	Primary Outcomes
NCT03342625 (BRIFU)	Sonalleve MRgFUS	15	Invasive ductal carcinoma	<1.5 cm	TBD	TBD	Resection at 1 mo	Evaluate thermal FUS with breast-specific ablation device and correlate findings with histologic criteria at 1 mo.
NCT03237572 (Breast 48)	Echopulse USgFUS	13	Confirmed metastatic or unresectable breast cancer	TBD	TBD	TBD	Biopsy at 1 mo	Thermal ablation will target 50% necrosis of primary tumor for combination with pembrolizumab in patients with metastatic disease. Change in proportion of CD8 + tumor-infiltrating lymphocytes (ratio CD8+/CD4+) in the primary ablation zone will be evaluated.
NCT05219695 (HMI)	HMIgFUSsystem	36	Invasive breast cancer: Stage 1	2–5 cm	TBD	TBD	Resection within 1 wk	Evaluate efficacy of new harmonic imaging technique for enhanced ultrasound feedback of lesion progression during treatment. Area of lesion shown in HMIgFUS will be compared to histology.

Abbreviations: TBD, to be determined; H&E, hematoxylin & eosin; MR-TI, magnetic resonance thermal imaging; DCE-MRI, dynamic contrast enhanced magnetic resonance imaging; MR-ARFI, magnetic resonance acoustic radiation force imaging.

Table 2
Summary of clinical investigations of focused ultrasound in breast fibroadenomas

Study Identifier	Device	Number of Patients	Size	Treatment Time	Ablation Success	Outcomes
Cavallo Marincola et al,[35] 2015	Model-JC HAIFU USgHIFU	10	2.65 cm	57.2 (40–100)	60	50% reduction in lesion diameter evaluated 3 mo post-treatment. Minor adverse pain in 2 patients.
Kovatcheva et al,[55] 2015	Echopulse USgFUS	42	3.9 cm^3	118 (60–255)	100	Superficial skin burn in 3 of 42 patients. 33.2% volumetric reduction at 3 mo, 59.2% at 6 mo, and 72.5% at 12 mo
Peek et al,[16] 2015; Peek et al,[21] 2018; Peek et al,[56] 2016	Echopulse USgFUS	20	7.3 cm^3	68.7	80	Evaluated circumferential ablation to reduce treatment time and confirmed 37.5% reduction compared to whole lesion ablation. 43.5% volumetric reduction at 6 mo. Pain completely resolved in 75% of patients.
Kovatcheva et al,[55] 2015	Echopulse USgFUS	20	1.82 cm^3/8.14 cm^3	60.6	100	20 patients with 26 FAs were grouped into either 1 FUS ($n = 19$) or 2 FUS ($n = 7$) treatments. Volume reduced at 1 mo, 3 mo, 1 y and a mean volume reduction of 77.3% (1 FUS) and 90.47% (2 FUS) was accomplished.
Peek et al,[16] 2015; Peek et al,[21] 2018; Peek et al,[56] 2016	Echopulse USgFUS	51	2.6 cm diameter	66	83	Circumferential ablation reduced treatment time by 29.4%. Volumetric reduction of 43.2% at 12 mo. Hyperpigmentation seen in 6 of 51 patients at 12 mo.

(continued on next page)

Table 2
(continued)

Study Identifier	Device	Number of Patients	Size	Treatment Time	Ablation Success	Outcomes
Hahn et al,[58] 2018	Echopulse USgFUS	27	1.08 cm³	80	96	Mean volume reduction of 61.6% at 6 mo and 84.8% at 12 mo. 86% of patients show no vital fibroadenoma cells in CNB at 12 mo. 74% of cases were assessed at total success.
Imankulov et al,[57] 2018	Model-JC HAIFU USgHIFU	40	N/A	N/A	100	HIFU (n = 40) was compared to partial resection (n = 40). 0% incidence of complication for HIFU compared to 20% for resection. Average hospital stay reduced by 52% with HIFU. Pain reduced by 44.7%.
Kwong et al,[54] 2021; Co et al,[60] 2022	Echopulse USgFUS	60	3.7 cm³	48.5/39.7/28.9	93	Treatment of 60 patients, 54 completed 12-mo follow-up. 3 cohorts were created to assess learning curve. Procedure time was significantly shorter for last 20 patients (P < .04). Mean tumor volume reduction in cohorts 1–3 were 45%, 51%, and 71%, respectively.

exhibit bruising, with these complications being self-resolving. Where opportunities are ripe to leverage FUS ablation routinely in the treatment of FAs, it is important to note that clinical user experience and learning curve is imperative. Indeed, Co and colleagues[60] tracked a single center's experience performing FUS for FA treatment over the first 60 patients and demonstrated significant improvement in achievement of lesion reduction in later cohorts, along with shortened treatment times—indicating improvement of outcomes after treating approximately 40 patients. Xiao and coinvestigators subsequently confirmed this finding by a cumulative sum analysis.[61] Additional trials will be needed to compare the impact and outcomes of FUS ablation to surgery or conservative management. As with MRgFUS ablation for breast malignancies, it is expected that advancements enabling lesion targeting and treatment monitoring will further the role of the technology for FAs.

Breast Cancer Metastases

While breast cancer is often diagnosed in early stages (90%–95%), approximately 20% to 30% of patients with primary breast cancer develop metastatic disease. The most common site of breast cancer metastasis is bone, which is involved in approximately 70% of all metastatic breast cancer cases. Indeed, 14% of patients with localized (stage I–III) breast cancer will develop bone metastases within 15 years of diagnosis. For patients suffering from breast cancer metastases to bone, rapid and durable pain relief is the clinical objective in their care. The primary palliative treatment of these patients has been external beam radiation, which offers improvement of pain control in 60% to 70% of patients. However, this palliation is often not durable, and its use of ionizing radiation limits the possibility of multiple treatments.

There is growing evidence for the utility of thermal ablation for palliation of pain associated with bone metastases, where the main objective for care is accomplished through periosteal nerve ablation and tumor debulking, both accomplished through thermal ablation ($>56°C$). MRgFUS is especially well suited for these ablations as it can mitigate the need for surgical interventions and lends favorably to repeat treatment where needed. Unlike soft tissue ablations, where the focal spot is well defined, leading to highly localized tissue heating, ablation of bone metastases with FUS is distinct as the absorption of sound waves by bone is greater than 50x compared to soft tissue. As a result, most of the energy accumulation is distributed on the bone–soft tissue interface.[62] Additionally, the presence of skeletal tissue results in a reduced ability to track treatment progress with real-time thermometry (MRgFUS) or changes in echogenicity (USgFUS). Despite these shortcomings, there is compelling evidence for the use of FUS for the treatment of breast metastases to bone due to growing empirical evidence of reduced pain and pain medication requirements following treatment.[63,64]

MRgFUS has been evaluated for nearly 20 years in the context of palliative care of bone metastases. In a retrospective study involving 13 patients, Catane and colleagues[65] reported no severe adverse events and significant improvement in visual analog scale pain score in radiotherapy refractory patients. A Phase III multicenter randomized controlled trial (147 patients) demonstrated that over 60% of patients experienced significant pain reduction at 3 months post-MRgFUS and 20% of patients reported complete pain relief.[66] In a recent report, Bongiovanni and colleagues[67] evaluated morphine equivalent daily dose (MEDD) scores following MRgFUS ablation and demonstrated a significant reduction from 37.5 to 7.3 mg by 30 days posttreatment. In a recent meta-analysis, Baal and colleagues[68] demonstrated that 55.8% of all patients no longer required pain medication following MRgFUS ablation of bone metastases, while an additional 33% were able to reduce drug intake.

Despite these obvious clinical successes, in a randomized controlled trial with 112 patients with FUS, Hurwitz and coinvestigators found that 56% of treatments reported adverse events, with 60% of those resolving on treatment day. The primary adverse events were postprocedural pain and skin burns likely resulting from noncompliance with treatment guidelines. It is important to further understand the heating and pain cessation mechanisms associated with MRgFUS for bone metastases as well as more rigorously characterize the extent of off-target heating to optimize acoustic parameters in future trials. Lee and colleagues[69] compared MRgFUS ablation to conventional radiotherapy in a matched-pair randomized controlled trial. Importantly, MRgFUS was shown to be significantly faster in providing pain relief compared to radiotherapy and showed no significant difference in pain response at 3 months. To this end, MRgFUS has been demonstrated to compete favorably with radiotherapy and other ablative techniques for this indication due to its noninvasive and nonionizing nature, spatial precision, repeatability, and availability of MR thermography feedback.[70]

Brain metastases occur in over 30% of breast cancers that express human epidermal growth factor receptor 2 (HER2). HER2 inhibitors (eg, trastuzumab) have shown promise in this patient subpopulation, but survival rates remain poor. The failure of systemically administered targeted therapies to cross the blood–brain barrier (BBB) places a significant constraint on therapeutic efficacy, suggesting a critical need for approaches to overcome this bottleneck in breast cancer metastases to the brain. MRgFUS, combined with systemically delivered, gas-filled microbubbles, has been employed to safely and transiently disrupt tumor-associated vasculature and the surrounding BBB to facilitate the delivery of systemic therapies into the brain across numerous pathologies including brain tumors.[71] Recently, a clinical trial (NCT03714243) demonstrated that MRgFUS confers enhancement of trastuzumab delivery to HER2+ breast cancer metastases to the brain. Meng and colleagues[72] summarized the results from a 4 patient trial that demonstrated a significant increase in radiolabeled trastuzumab via single-photon emission computed tomography (SPECT) imaging—offering the first visual demonstration of a monoclonal antibody being delivered across the BBB with FUS. No adverse events were noted. While lesion volume changes were noted in these patients, interpretations were limited by small sample size, variability in follow-up, and lack of blinding—necessitating a larger follow-on trial in the future.

Notably, the incidence of breast cancer metastasis to the liver is also high. The liver represents the third most common site of metastasis behind bone and lungs, often associated with more aggressive phenotypes and worse prognoses.[73] An ongoing clinical trial in Norway is leveraging the improved oxygenation and augmented drug delivery resulting from FUS and microbubbles for treatment of breast metastases to the liver (NCT03477019). The proof-of-concept established by these novel trials will set the stage for the increased study of MRgFUS in the treatment of brain and liver metastases in patients with breast cancer. **Table 3** provides a complete overview of the clinical trials investigating MRgFUS in breast cancer metastases.

LOOKING AHEAD

The last 2 decades have seen astonishing growth in applications of FUS for breast tumor care (**Fig. 4**). Early trials were primarily centered on achieving maximal ablation in primary breast tumors, both benign and malignant. In this regard, issues that remain for wider clinical adoption include the duration of treatment times (particularly in association with MRgFUS procedures compared to USgFUS), uncertainty of margin status in the absence of excision or multimodality care, and persistence of palpable masses (fat necrosis) that can occur in a minority of patients after ablation. It is expected that these issues can be surmounted with further consideration to technical improvement of new or existing image-guided FUS devices, deployment of additional rigorously designed clinical investigations, and continued consideration to where FUS ablation rests within the current surgical paradigm for breast tumors.

In acknowledgment of the multimodal nature of breast cancer care, it is also worth highlighting that FUS has also been combined with the mainstays of chemotherapy and radiotherapy in clinical settings, bringing to bear paradigms for FUS requiring distinct sonication techniques from those set forth for maximal thermal ablation. For example, a recent Phase I trial deployed MRgFUS for hyperthermia in combination with ThermoDox in patients with de novo stage IV breast cancer—demonstrating that hyperthermia aids the intravascular release of doxorubicin from ThermoDox more favorably over ThermoDox or conventional doxorubicin alone.[19] MRgFUS has also been deployed in combination with microbubbles for radiosensitization of breast cancers, with results from a recent Phase I prospective trial demonstrating the safety of combining FUS and fractionated external beam radiotherapy in patients with gross unresected disease.[74] Together, these and other emerging studies highlight the opportunities for FUS as a powerful complement to the current standard of care for breast cancers.

In 2017, a "first-in-human" clinical trial launched to investigate combination of FUS thermal ablation with immunotherapy (pembrolizumab; Keytruda) in patients with metastatic breast cancer (NCT03237572). In the interest of leveraging FUS to augment antigen presentation and immune specificity of checkpoint blockade, this trial was designed with a subtotal (up to 50% of the tumor) ablation schema intended to preserve regions of intact, yet immunogenic primary tumor tissue to support mobilization of a systemic immune response. Similarly, subtotal thermal ablation with FUS is currently being tested in combination with low-dose gemcitabine in a "treat-and-resect" trial examining immunologic control in early-stage breast cancers (NCT04796220). Taken together, these studies underscore the adaptability of FUS techniques based on the unique considerations for novel therapeutic combinations. The unparalleled versatility of FUS technology offers a promising outlook for growing applications of the technology beyond ablation.

Table 3
Summary of clinical investigations of focused ultrasound in breast cancer metastases

Study Identifier	Site	Cases	Imaging Guidance/Device	Outcomes
Liberman et al,[78] 2009	Bone	31	MRgFUS/Exablate 2000	Pain prescore of 5.9 which was reduced at 3 d to 3.8 and at 3 mo to 1.8; complete response (CR) noted in 36% of patients and opioid reduction in 67% of patients
Catane et al,[65] 2007	Bone	13	MRgFUS/Exablate 2000	Average pain prescore 5.5, which reduced at 3 d to 2.3 and at 3 mo to 0.3; No significant adverse events
Napoli et al,[64] 2013	Bone	18	MRgFUS/Exablate 2000	Pain prescore of 7.1 which reduced to 2.5 at 1 mo and 1.0 at 3 mo, CR in 72% of patients evaluated at 3 mo, 72% patients discontinued medicine at 3 mo. Quality of life (QOL) prescore: 4.8 which improved to 0.5 at 3 mo.
Hurwitz et al,[66] 2014	Bone	112	MRgFUS/Exablate 2000	CR of 23.2% determined at 3 mo; mean reduction in pain scale of 3.6 for FUS and 0.7 for placebo. 27% patients discontinued pain medicine at 3 mo. QOL has 2.4 point superior to placebo at 3 mo. 60.3% of adverse events (AE) resolved on treatment day.
Gu et al,[70] 2015	Bone	23	MRgFUS/Exablate 2000	Pain prescore of 6.0 which reduced to 3.7 at 1 wk and 2.2 at 3 mo, QOL improved from 39 pretreatment to 26 1 and 213 mo post-treatment.
Lee et al,[69] 2017	Bone	63	MRgFUS/Exablate 2000	FUS was compared to radiotherapy (RT), no significant difference in MEDD for RT vs FUS. Pain prescore 6.2 and 6.6 for RT and FUS, respectively, which reduced to 2.5 after 1 wk post-FUS and 4.8 1 wk post-RT
Bertrand et al,[79] 2018	Bone	17	MRgFUS/Exablate 2000	Pain prescore of 7.5 which reduced to 1.9 at 1 mo post-FUS. 38% CR and 50% PR, 270.6 Morphine equivalent daily dose (MEDD) pre-FUS which reduced to 113.75 after 1 mo.
Bongiovanni et al,[67] 2022	Bone	12	MRgFUS/Exablate 2000	50% CR at 30 d, pretreatment MEDD of 37.5 mg which reduced to 14.3 mg after 7 d and 7.3 mg after 1 mo. QOL prescore of 40 (QLQ-C15-PAL) which improved to 73.3 1 mo post-FUS. 1 grade 2 skin burn
Hsu et al,[80] 2022	Bone	20	MRgFUS/Exablate 2000	80% CR evaluated at 3 mo and 67.7%; overall radiographic response rate at 3 mo.
NCT03714243 (BBBD)	Brain	10	MRgFUS/Exablate 4000 Type 2 Neurosystem	Result of first 4 patients published in Meng et al. Patients will undergo up to 6 study treatment cycles every 2–3 wk. Follow-up will be tracked for 12 wk following last treatment
NCT02307612	Liver	17	Clinical ultrasound scanner	Evaluation of sonopermeation and potential for therapeutic response to chemotherapy to be improved by FUS

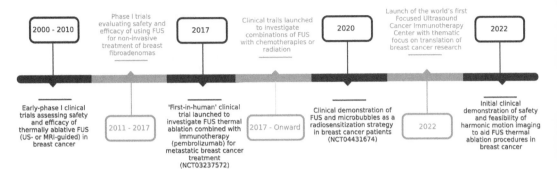

Fig. 4. Timeline overviewing notable milestones in clinical development landscape for breast tumor intervention with FUS. (Created with Biorender.com.)

SUMMARY

In conclusion, the evolution and expanding clinical application of FUS technologies, particularly MRgFUS, reflect a paradigm shift toward less invasive intervention in benign and malignant breast tumor settings. This review summarizes the significant advancements in FUS technology and mounting clinical evidence for its utility as a breast tumor intervention. The highlighted applications also demonstrate the technology's versatility, which presently ranges from thermally ablative debulking of primary and benign breast lesions to direct targeting of distal metastases for palliation or adjunct therapy. Owing to advances in MR imaging technology, MRgFUS elevates this noninvasive treatment option to one that also affords precise treatment planning, real-time monitoring, and acute outcome evaluation, aligning with the goals of personalized and patient-centered care. As the field continues to demonstrate the full potential of FUS in breast oncology, it is imperative to address current limitations, including the high cost and technical demands of MRgFUS, to ensure broader accessibility and adoption. USgFUS offers potential benefits for simplified and potentially lower cost treatments but presently lacks the aforementioned feedback mechanisms that would be key to precise, feedback-controlled interventions. To date, clinical investigation of USgFUS systems has also been limited to thermal ablation—in contrast with the more diverse portfolio of investigations leveraging MRgFUS. Nonetheless, future research should focus on optimizing treatment protocols and expanding clinical indications for both classes of FUS devices. The rapidly expanding exploration of this space, ranging from development of novel clinical devices to novel combinatory approaches (eg, combination with immunotherapy for systemic disease control[75]), affirms the promise of FUS as a disruptive technology for breast tumor care—one that could conceivably shift the paradigm for the current standard of care and enable noninvasive, targeted intervention to become a cornerstone of clinical breast tumor treatment.

CLINICS CARE POINTS

- Breast tumors (benign and malignant) remain a global health burden, and traditional surgery is not ideal due to its invasive nature.

- FUS offers an exciting noninvasive, nonionizing strategy for focal interventions in breast FAs, primary breast cancers, and select sites of metastasis.

- Investigational and commercial systems are now available for both MR and ultrasound imaging-guided FUS, offering distinct strengths and weaknesses for treatment planning, real-time monitoring, and procedure duration.

- Applications for FUS thermal ablation in primary breast tumors have burgeoned over the last 2 decades, and more recently emerging are applications for palliation of bone metastases. There is strong evidence for the safety, feasibility, and patient satisfaction associated with these applications.

- Promising new clinical applications on the horizon for FUS in breast malignancies include combinatorial approaches with small molecule chemotherapy, radiotherapy (radiosensitization), or immunotherapy, as well as BBB opening for targeted therapeutic delivery to brain metastases.

DISCLOSURE

The work of N.D. Sheybani was supported by funding from the National Institutes of Health Director's Early Independence Award (DP5OD031846) and

Wallace H. Coulter Center for Translational Research. The work of Z.E.F. Demir was supported by an NIH Cancer Training Grant (T32 CA009109).

REFERENCES

1. Hong R, Xu B. Breast cancer: an up-to-date review and future perspectives. Cancer Commun 2022;42: 913–36.

2. Kashyap D, Pal D, Sharma R, et al. Global increase in breast cancer incidence: risk factors and preventive measures. BioMed Res Int 2022;2022:9605439.

3. Siegel RL, Giaquinto AN, Jemal A. Cancer statistics, 2024. CA A Cancer J Clin 2024;74(1):12–49.

4. Wilkinson L, Gathani T. Understanding breast cancer as a global health concern. The British Journal of Radiology 2022;95:20211033.

5. Jagannathan G, White MJ, Xian RR, et al. A new landscape of testing and therapeutics in metastatic breast cancer. Clin Lab Med 2023;43:299–321.

6. Brenin DR. Ablative Treatment of Breast Cancer; Are We There Yet? Current Breast Cancer Reports 2019; 11:43–50.

7. Bailey M, Khokhlova V, Sapozhnikov O, et al. Physical mechanisms of the therapeutic effect of ultrasound (a review). Acoust Phys 2003;49:369–88.

8. Salomir R, Vimeux FC, de Zwart JA, et al. Hyperthermia by MR-guided focused ultrasound: accurate temperature control based on fast MRI and a physical model of local energy deposition and heat conduction. Magn Reson Med 2000;43:342–7.

9. Zhu L, Altman MB, Laszlo A, et al. Ultrasound hyperthermia technology for radiosensitization. Ultrasound Med Biol 2019;45:1025–43.

10. Xu Z, Hall TL, Vlaisavljevich E, et al. the first noninvasive, non-ionizing, non-thermal ablation technique based on ultrasound. Int J Hyperther 2021;38: 561–75.

11. Khokhlova VA, Fowlkes JB, Roberts WW, et al. Histotripsy methods in mechanical disintegration of tissue: Towards clinical applications. Int J Hyperther 2015;31:145–62.

12. Vidal-Jove J, Serres X, Vlaisavljevich E, et al. First-in-man histotripsy of hepatic tumors: the THERESA trial, a feasibility study. Int J Hyperther 2022;39: 1115–23.

13. Hendricks-Wenger A, Hutchison R, Vlaisavljevich E, et al. Immunological effects of histotripsy for cancer therapy. Frontiers in oncology 2021;11:681629.

14. Osada T, Jiang X, Zhao Y, et al. The use of histotripsy as intratumoral immunotherapy beyond tissue ablation—the rationale for exploring the immune effects of histotripsy. Int J Hyperther 2023;40: 2263672.

15. Timbie KF, Mead BP, Price RJ. Drug and gene delivery across the blood–brain barrier with focused ultrasound. J Contr Release 2015;219:61–75.

16. Peek M, Ahmed M, Napoli A, et al. Systematic review of high-intensity focused ultrasound ablation in the treatment of breast cancer. Journal of British Surgery 2015;102:873–82.

17. Schmitz A, Gianfelice D, Daniel B, et al. Image-guided focused ultrasound ablation of breast cancer: current status, challenges, and future directions. Eur Radiol 2008;18:1431–41.

18. Lyon PC, Griffiths LF, Lee J, et al. Clinical trial protocol for TARDOX: a phase I study to investigate the feasibility of targeted release of lyso-thermosensitive liposomal doxorubicin (ThermoDox®) using focused ultrasound in patients with liver tumours. Journal of therapeutic ultrasound 2017;5:1–8.

19. de Maar JS, Suelmann BBM, Braat MNGJA, et al. Phase I feasibility study of Magnetic Resonance guided High Intensity Focused Ultrasound-induced hyperthermia, Lyso-Thermosensitive Liposomal Doxorubicin and cyclophosphamide in de novo stage IV breast cancer patients: study protocol of the i-GO study. BMJ Open 2020;10:e040162.

20. Foley JL, Eames M, Snell J, et al. Image-guided focused ultrasound: state of the technology and the challenges that lie ahead. Imag Med 2013;5:357.

21. Peek MC, Wu F. High-intensity focused ultrasound in the treatment of breast tumours. Ecancermedicalscience 2018;12.

22. Huber PE, Jenne JW, Rastert R, et al. A new noninvasive approach in breast cancer therapy using magnetic resonance imaging-guided focused ultrasound surgery. Cancer Res 2001;61:8441–7.

23. Dick E, Gedroyc W. ExAblate® magnetic resonance-guided focused ultrasound system in multiple body applications. Expet Rev Med Dev 2010;7:589–97.

24. Feril LB, Fernan RL, Tachibana K. High-intensity focused ultrasound in the treatment of breast cancer. Curr Med Chem 2021;28:5179–88.

25. Knuttel FM, Huijsse SEM, Feenstra TL, et al. Early health technology assessment of magnetic resonance-guided high intensity focused ultrasound ablation for the treatment of early-stage breast cancer. Journal of therapeutic ultrasound 2017;5:1–10.

26. Deckers R, Merckel LG, Denis de Senneville B, et al. Performance analysis of a dedicated breast MR-HIFU system for tumor ablation in breast cancer patients. Phys Med Biol 2015;60:5527.

27. Karzova MM, Kreider W, Partanen A, et al. Comparative Characterization of Nonlinear Ultrasound Fields Generated by Sonalleve V1 and V2 MR-HIFU Systems. IEEE Trans Ultrason Ferroelectrics Freq Control 2023;70(6):521–37.

28. Ellis S, Rieke V, Kohi M, et al. Clinical applications for magnetic resonance guided high intensity focused ultrasound (MRgHIFU): present and future. Journal of medical imaging and radiation oncology 2013; 57:391–9.

29. Ebbini ES, Ter Haar G. Ultrasound-guided therapeutic focused ultrasound: Current status and future directions. Int J Hyperther 2015;31:77–89.

30. Wu F, Wang ZB, Chen WZ, et al. Extracorporeal high intensity focused ultrasound ablation in the treatment of 1038 patients with solid carcinomas in China: an overview. Ultrason Sonochem 2004;11:149–54.

31. Gianfelice D, Khiat A, Amara M, et al. MR imaging–guided focused US ablation of breast cancer: histopathologic assessment of effectiveness—initial experience. Radiology 2003;227:849–55.

32. Gianfelice D, Khiat A, Boulanger Y, et al. Feasibility of magnetic resonance imaging–guided focused ultrasound surgery as an adjunct to tamoxifen therapy in high-risk surgical patients with breast carcinoma. J Vasc Intervent Radiol 2003;14:1275–82.

33. Furusawa H, Namba K, Thomsen S, et al. Magnetic resonance–guided focused ultrasound surgery of breast cancer: reliability and effectiveness. J Am Coll Surg 2006;203:54–63.

34. Furusawa H, Namba K, Nakahara H, et al. The evolving non-surgical ablation of breast cancer: MR guided focused ultrasound (MRgFUS). Breast cancer 2007;14:55–8.

35. Cavallo Marincola B, Pediconi F, Anzidei M, et al. High-intensity focused ultrasound in breast pathology: non-invasive treatment of benign and malignant lesions. Expet Rev Med Dev 2015;12:191–9.

36. Merckel LG, Bartels LW, Köhler MO, et al. MR-guided high-intensity focused ultrasound ablation of breast cancer with a dedicated breast platform. Cardiovascular and interventional radiology 2013;36:292–301.

37. Merckel LG, Knuttel FM, Deckers R, et al. First clinical experience with a dedicated MRI-guided high-intensity focused ultrasound system for breast cancer ablation. Eur Radiol 2016;26:4037–46.

38. Adams-Tew SI, Johnson S, Odéen H, et al. Validation of a drift-corrected 3D MR temperature imaging sequence for breast MR-guided focused ultrasound treatments. Magn Reson Imag 2023;96:126–34.

39. Coon J, Payne A, Roemer R. HIFU treatment time reduction in superficial tumours through focal zone path selection. Int J Hyperther 2011;27:465–81.

40. Payne A, Merrill R, Minalga E, et al. A breast-specific MR guided focused ultrasound platform and treatment protocol: first-in-human technical evaluation. IEEE (Inst Electr Electron Eng) Trans Biomed Eng 2020;68:893–904.

41. Diakite M, Odéen H, Todd N, et al. Toward real-time temperature monitoring in fat and aqueous tissue during magnetic resonance–guided high-intensity focused ultrasound using a three-dimensional proton resonance frequency T1 method. Magn Reson Med 2014;72:178–87.

42. Wu F, Wang ZB, Cao YD, et al. A randomised clinical trial of high-intensity focused ultrasound ablation for the treatment of patients with localised breast cancer. British journal of cancer 2003;89:2227–33.

43. Wu F, Wang ZB, Cao YD, et al. Heat fixation of cancer cells ablated with high-intensity–focused ultrasound in patients with breast cancer. Am J Surg 2006;192:179–84.

44. Wu F, Wang ZB, Zhu H, et al. Extracorporeal high intensity focused ultrasound treatment for patients with breast cancer. Breast Cancer Res Treat 2005;92:51–60.

45. Kim SH, Jung SE, Kim HL, et al. The potential role of dynamic MRI in assessing the effectiveness of high-intensity focused ultrasound ablation of breast cancer. Int J Hyperther 2010;26:594–603.

46. Guan L, Xu G. Damage effect of high-intensity focused ultrasound on breast cancer tissues and their vascularities. World J Surg Oncol 2016;14:1–17.

47. Maleke C, Konofagou EE. Harmonic motion imaging for focused ultrasound (HMIFU): a fully integrated technique for sonication and monitoring of thermal ablation in tissues. Phys Med Biol 2008;53:1773.

48. Curiel L, Hynynen K. Localized harmonic motion imaging for focused ultrasound surgery targeting. Ultrasound Med Biol 2011;37:1230–9.

49. Lewis MA, Staruch RM, Chopra R. Thermometry and ablation monitoring with ultrasound. Int J Hyperther 2015;31:163–81.

50. Gonnah AR, Masoud O, AbdelWahab M, et al. The Role of High Intensity Focused Ultrasound in the Treatment of Fibroadenomas: A Systematic Review. Breast Care 2023;18:278–87.

51. Stachs A, Stubert J, Reimer T, et al. Benign breast disease in women. Deutsches Ärzteblatt International 2019;116:565.

52. Klinger K, Bhimani C, Shames J, et al. Fibroadenoma: from imaging evaluation to treatment. J Am Osteopath Coll Radiol 2019;8:17–30.

53. Akin IB, Balci P. Fibroadenomas: a multidisciplinary review of the variants. Clin Imag 2021;71:83–100.

54. Kwong A, Co M, Chen C, et al. Prospective clinical trial on high-intensity focused ultrasound for the treatment of breast fibroadenoma. Breast J 2021;27:294–6.

55. Kovatcheva R, Guglielmina JN, Abehsera M, et al. Ultrasound-guided high-intensity focused ultrasound treatment of breast fibroadenoma—a multicenter experience. Journal of therapeutic ultrasound 2015;3:1–8.

56. Peek M, Ahmed M, Scudder J, et al. High intensity focused ultrasound in the treatment of breast fibroadenomata: results of the HIFU-F trial. Int J Hyperther 2016;32:881–8.

57. Imankulov S, Tuganbekov T, Razbadauskas A, et al. HIFU treatment for fibroadenoma-a clinical study at National Scientific Research Centre, Astana, Kazakhstan. JPMA. The Journal of the Pakistan Medical Association 2018;68:1378–80.

58. Hahn M, Fugunt R, Schoenfisch B, et al. High intensity focused ultrasound (HIFU) for the treatment of symptomatic breast fibroadenoma. Int J Hyperther 2018;35:463–70.

59. Hynynen K, Pomeroy O, Smith DN, et al. MR imaging-guided focused ultrasound surgery of fibroadenomas in the breast: a feasibility study. Radiology 2001;219:176–85.

60. Co M, Chen C, Lee C, et al. Prospective clinical trial on the learning curve of high-intensity-focused ultrasound for the treatment of breast fibroadenoma. Surg Today 2022;1-6.

61. Xiao Y, Liang M, Chen M, et al. Evaluating the learning curve of high intensity focus ultrasound for breast fibroadenoma by CUSUM analysis: a multicenter study. Int J Hyperther 2022;39:1238–44.

62. Scipione R, Anzidei M, Bazzocchi A, et al. HIFU for Bone Metastases and other Musculoskeletal Applications. Semin Intervent Radiol 2018;35(4):261–7.

63. Chan M, Dennis K, Huang Y, et al. Magnetic Resonance–Guided High-Intensity-Focused Ultrasound for Palliation of Painful Skeletal Metastases: A Pilot Study. Technol Cancer Res Treat 2017;16:570–6.

64. Napoli A, Anzidei M, Marincola BC, et al. Primary pain palliation and local tumor control in bone metastases treated with magnetic resonance-guided focused ultrasound. Invest Radiol 2013;48:351–8.

65. Catane R, Beck A, Inbar Y, et al. MR-guided focused ultrasound surgery (MRgFUS) for the palliation of pain in patients with bone metastases—preliminary clinical experience. Ann Oncol 2007;18:163–7.

66. Hurwitz MD, Ghanouni P, Kanaev SV, et al. Magnetic resonance–guided focused ultrasound for patients with painful bone metastases: phase III trial results. Journal of the National Cancer Institute 2014;106: dju082.

67. Bongiovanni A, Foca F, Oboldi D, et al. 3-T magnetic resonance–guided high-intensity focused ultrasound (3 T-MR-HIFU) for the treatment of pain from bone metastases of solid tumors. Support Care Cancer 2022;30:5737–45.

68. Baal JD, Chen WC, Baal U, et al. Efficacy and safety of magnetic resonance-guided focused ultrasound for the treatment of painful bone metastases: a systematic review and meta-analysis. Skeletal Radiol 2021;50:2459–69.

69. Lee H-L, Kuo CC, Tsai JT, et al. Magnetic resonance-guided focused ultrasound versus conventional radiation therapy for painful bone metastasis: a matched-pair study. JBJS 2017;99:1572–8.

70. Gu J, Wang H, Tang N, et al. Magnetic resonance guided focused ultrasound surgery for pain palliation of bone metastases: early experience of clinical application in China. Zhonghua Yixue Zazhi 2015; 95:3328–32.

71. Arvanitis CD, Askoxylakis V, Guo Y, et al. Mechanisms of enhanced drug delivery in brain metastases with focused ultrasound-induced blood–tumor barrier disruption. Proc Natl Acad Sci USA 2018; 115:E8717–26.

72. Meng Y, Reilly RM, Pezo RC, et al. MR-guided focused ultrasound enhances delivery of trastuzumab to Her2-positive brain metastases. Sci Transl Med 2021;13:eabj4011.

73. Tsilimigras DI, Brodt P, Clavien PA, et al. Liver metastases. Nat Rev Dis Prim 2021;7:27.

74. Dasgupta A, Saifuddin M, McNabb E, et al. Novel MRI-guided Focussed Ultrasound Stimulated Microbubble Radiation Enhancement Treatment for Breast Cancer. Sci Rep 2023;13(1):13566.

75. Sheybani ND, Price RJ. Perspectives on recent progress in focused ultrasound immunotherapy. Theranostics 2019;9:7749.

76. Zippel DB, Papa MZ. The use of MR imaging guided focused ultrasound in breast cancer patients; a preliminary phase one study and review. Breast Cancer 2005;12(1):32–8.

77. Khiat A, Gianfelice D, Amara M, Boulanger Y. Influence of post-treatment delay on the evaluation of the response to focused ultrasound surgery of breast cancer by dynamic contrast enhanced MRI. Br J Radiol 2006;79(940):308–14.

78. Liberman B, Gianfelice D, Inbar Y, et al. Pain palliation in patients with bone metastases using MR-guided focused ultrasound surgery: a multicenter study. Ann Surg Oncol 2009;16(1):140–6.

79. Bertrand AS, Iannessi A, Natale R, et al. Focused ultrasound for the treatment of bone metastases: effectiveness and feasibility. J Ther Ultrasound 2018;6:8.

80. Hsu FC, Lee HL, Chen YJ, et al. A Few-Shot Learning Approach Assists in the Prognosis Prediction of Magnetic Resonance-Guided Focused Ultrasound for the Local Control of Bone Metastatic Lesions. Cancers (Basel) 2022;14(2):445.

Magnetic Resonance–Guided Focused Ultrasound Surgery for Gynecologic Indications

Elisabeth R. Knorren, MD[a,b,*], Ingrid M. Nijholt, PhD[a],
Joke M. Schutte, MD, PhD[b], Martijn F. Boomsma, MD, PhD[a,c]

KEYWORDS

- MRI • Focused ultrasound surgery • MRgFUS • Gynecologic indications

KEY POINTS

- Magnetic resonance–guided focused ultrasound surgery (MRgFUS) is a promising technique for the treatment of uterine fibroids, uterine adenomyosis, abdominal wall endometriosis, and painful recurrent gynecologic malignancies, offering the advantages of noninvasive therapy and preservation of fertility.
- Prospective comparative cohort studies or randomized controlled trials are needed to establish long-term (cost)effectiveness compared to standard care before clinical implementation can take place.
- Reimbursement and controlled implementation are needed to establish widespread adoption of MRgFUS in gynecology and open up opportunities to expand the range of gynecologic indications for MRgFUS.

INTRODUCTION

Magnetic resonance–guided focused ultrasound surgery (MRgFUS) has been increasingly used in medicine since the early 2000s.[1] MRgFUS uses high-intensity ultrasound beams focused by a focused ultrasound surgery (FUS) transducer to ablate target tissue under real-time magnetic resonance (MR) monitoring of the target and surrounding tissues.[1] (Fig. 1) Especially in benign gynecologic diseases, there is a growing demand for noninvasive, nonhormonal, and fertility-preserving treatment options such as MRgFUS.[2] Technical success of the MRgFUS treatment is assessed as non-perfused volume (NPV) by T1-weighted gadolinium-contrast MRI. The NPV ratio

(NPV%) is the ratio between the NPV and the pretreatment volume of the target tissue.[1]

Hitherto, several gynecologic indications have been treated with MRgFUS: uterine fibroids (UFs), uterine adenomyosis (UA), abdominal wall endometriosis (AWE), and palliative treatment of painful recurrent gynecologic malignancies (PRGMs). This review provides an overview per indication of the following outcomes: screening methods, volume reduction, symptom reduction (measured by validated questionnaires on symptoms as transformed symptom severity score [tSSS], health-related quality of life [HRQoL], and pain scores [0–10]), complications, reintervention rates, reproductive outcomes, and costs.

[a] Department of Radiology, Isala Hospital, Dokter van Heesweg 2, 8025 AB, Zwolle, the Netherlands;
[b] Department of Obstetrics and Gynecology, Isala Hospital, Dokter van Heesweg 2, 8025 AB, Zwolle, the Netherlands; [c] Imaging & Oncology Division, Image Sciences Institute, University Medical Center Utrecht, Heidelberglaan 100, 3584 CX, Utrecht, the Netherlands
* Corresponding author. Isala Hospital, Dokter van Heesweg 2, 8025 AB, Zwolle, the Netherlands.
E-mail address: e.r.knorren@isala.nl

Magn Reson Imaging Clin N Am 32 (2024) 615–628
https://doi.org/10.1016/j.mric.2024.02.005
1064-9689/24/© 2024 Elsevier Inc. All rights reserved.

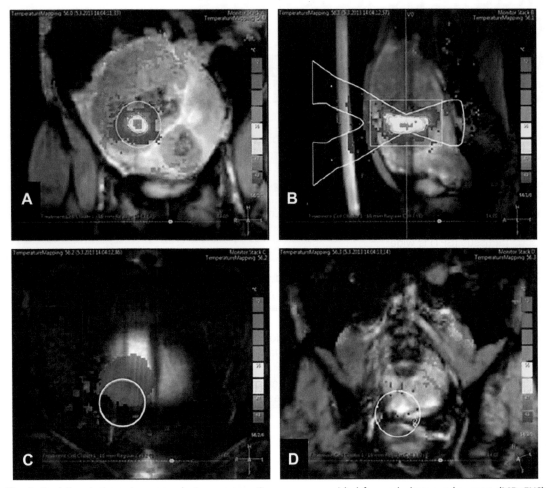

Fig. 1. Real-time temperature map during a magnetic resonance–guided focused ultrasound surgery (MRgFUS) sonication in a target fibroid (*A, B*), skin (*C*), and near-filed and far-field heating (*D*). (*Courtesy* of Inez Verpalen, MD PhD, Amsterdam, Netherlands.)

METHODS

Systematic literature searches were conducted in PubMed/MEDLINE and Cochrane databases for each indication. English full-text publications from peer-reviewed journals were included, if they reported on at least 1 of our outcomes. The level of evidence (LoE) according to the Oxford Center of Evidence-Based Medicine 2011 and the grade of recommendation (GoR) were determined per outcome. LoE 1 and GoR A indicate reliable evidence that can be used in clinical practice. LoE 5 and GoR D indicate inconclusive evidence that provides only a suggestion for clinical practice.[3,4] (Appendix 1 – Tables 1 and 2) The data in this review are based on publications with the highest LoE available. Data of systematic reviews were supplemented with more recent literature when these were not included in the systematic review.

UTERINE FIBROIDS

UFs are the most common benign tumors of the female reproductive organs. Approximately 25% of reproductive women have symptomatic UFs.[5] Symptoms include menorrhagia, dysmenorrhea, mechanical complaints or subfertility, depending on UF size and location. Pharmacologic treatment consists of tranexamic acid often combined with nonsteroidal anti-inflammatory drugs or hormonal therapy as oral contraceptives, intrauterine devices or gonadotropin-releasing hormone analogues. When pharmacologic treatment is inadequate, inappropriate, or not preferred by the patient, (minimally) invasive treatments such as hysteroscopic myomectomy, uterine artery embolization (UAE), surgical myomectomy, or hysterectomy are alternatives. UFs were the first indication for which MRgFUS was approved by the Food and Drugs Administration in 2004, and are therefore the best-studied gynecologic indication for MRgFUS.[1]

Screening

Not every UF is suitable for MRgFUS. A screening MRI is performed to determine eligibility. Eligibility criteria can be divided into anatomic and MRI characteristics (**Table 1**) (**Fig. 2**).

Pedunculated, subserosal UFs are often ineligible due to the risk of separation of the UF from the stalk, and cervical UFs are often ineligible due to pubic bone interference. Submucosal UFs and intracavitary UFs are often ineligible due to the risk of prolonged vaginal necrotic discharge after MRgFUS or vaginal expulsion.[6] When subcutaneous fat tissue (SFT) is wider than 4 cm, there is a risk of thermal injury to the SFT due to near-field heating and insufficient heating of the target tissue because of lower specific heat capacity, lower conductivity, and lower perfusion of the SFT.[7] Furthermore, sonications can be created until approximately 10 cm, so the entire UF should be within this range. Manipulation techniques can be applied to increase eligibility.[8]

Screening tools based on MRI characteristics are typically based on T2-weighted signal intensity (SI) of the UF, with the Funaki classification as the most used tool.[9] Hypointense and isointense UFs (Funaki 1&2) are considered eligible for MRgFUS, whereas hyperintense UFs (Funaki 3) are not, presumably due to high fluid load or perfusion of these tissues, resulting in insufficient heating.[9] However, UFs greater than 10 cm or Funaki 3 UFs with heterogeneous SI can benefit from pretreatment with gonadotropin-releasing hormone analogues, as this shrinks the UF and optimizes sonication efficiency, making these UFs eligible for MRgFUS after all.[10] Research has shown that multiparametric MRI parameters can distinguish UFs from myometrium and can discriminate UF tissue types, potentially predicting MRgFUS outcomes.[11] However, these parameters have not yet been implemented in screening tools for clinical use. As eligibility for MRgFUS treatment is based on multiple interacting factors whose individual contribution to a successful treatment is not yet fully understood, each case must be evaluated individually.

Non-perfused Volume Ratio

In the early days of MRgFUS for UFs, restrictive treatment protocols aiming for NPV% of 30% to 40% were used for safety reasons. This restriction was released when research showed that higher NPV% could be achieved safely and was associated with greater clinical success.[12] Nowadays, unrestrictive MRgFUS protocols are standard practice. Therefore, our UF overview is based on publications with unrestricted MRgFUS protocols. When these were not available, results of studies with restricted treatment protocols are presented.

Bitton and colleagues (2023)[13] suggested another parameter to predict clinical success: the ratio of NPV to total fibroid load (TFL). Increasing NPV/TFL ratios showed significantly better treatment outcomes. This ratio may provide a better prediction of clinical outcomes than the NPV% due to inclusion of non-targeted and possibly symptom-contributing UFs and should therefore be reported together with NPV% in future studies of MRgFUS for UFs to determine its predictive value.[14]

Volume and Symptom Reduction

A systematic review by Verpalen and colleagues[15] included 18 publications covering 16 studies with 1418 patients that were treated with unrestrictive MRgFUS. They reported a pooled mean NPV% (95% confidence interval (CI)) of 68.1% (59.9–76.3), with a pooled mean volume reduction of 33.2% (27.9–38.5), 36.6% (28.9–44.3), and 37.7% (32.7–42.8) at 3, 6, and 12 months follow-up, respectively. tSSS decreased by 43.0% (95%CI 34.3–51.7), 49.3% (95%CI 40.0–58.5), and 59.9% (95%CI 53.7–66.1) at 3, 6, and 12 months follow-up, respectively. HRQoL scores improved by 31.4% (95%CI -16.3–79.2) and

---

Table 1
Eligibility criteria for magnetic resonance–guided focused ultrasound surgery for uterine fibroids according to anatomic and MRI characteristics

Anatomic Characteristics	MRI Characteristics
• Intramural or subserosal UF • SFT<4 cm • Dorsal side of UF < 10 cm of abdominal wall • Size UF > 2 and < 10 cm	• Hypointense/isointense signal intensity of UF on T2w MRI compared to myometrium (eg, Funaki) • Homogeneous contrast enhancement on T1w MRI

Abbreviations: SFT, subcutaneous fat tissue; T1w, T1-weighted; T2w, T2-weighted; UF, uterine fibroid.

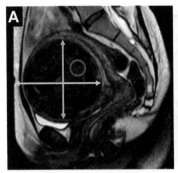 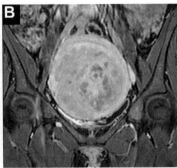 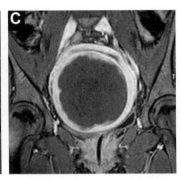

Fig. 2. Inclusion criteria for magnetic resonance–guided focused ultrasound surgery (MRgFUS) for uterine fibroids (UF) based on anatomic and MRI characteristics. (*A*) Sagittal T2-weighted MRI with UF positioned mainly intramural of anterior uterine wall. Blue arrow indicates maximum diameter of UF less than 10 cm, green arrow indicates dorsal side of UF less than 10 cm of the abdominal wall, yellow asterisk indicates subcutaneous fat tissue less than 4 cm, red circle indicates signal intensity of the UF compared to the myometrium. (*B*) Coronal T1-weighted post-gadolinium MRI with almost homogeneous contrast enhancement before MRgFUS. (*C*) Coronal T1-weighted post-gadolinium MRI immediately after MRgFUS showing a non-perfused volume ratio of 99%.

31.5% (95%CI -5.6–68.5) at 3 and 6 months follow-up, respectively. After the review by Verpalen and colleagues, 4 studies (2 prospective cohorts n = 288 and 43, 2 retrospective cohorts n = 16 and 33) were published on symptom improvement after unrestrictive MRgFUS.[16–19] Three studies reported mean NPV% of 71.0% to 89.8% (range) and 1 study (n = 33) reported median NPV% of 89.8% (interquartile range, 29.9%). Two studies reported mean volume reduction 3 months after treatment of 27% (n = 288) and 45.6% (n = 16), respectively, and 2 studies reported mean volume reduction 6 months after MRgFUS of 39% (n = 288) and 59.1% (n = 43). One study (n = 33) reported median volume reduction of 36.9% 6 months after MRgFUS. Two studies reported tSSS improvement 6 months after MRgFUS of 54.9% (mean, n = 43) and 66.5% (median, n = 33). In 1 study (n = 288) patients reported their quality of life at 3 and 6 months better in 61% and 53%, and much better in 8% and 23%, respectively. Another study (n = 16) reported improvement of mean HRQoL of 41.5%, 43.3%, and 33.3% at 3, 6, and 12 months, respectively.

Complications

In the systematic review and meta-analysis by Verpalen and colleagues,[15] complications were reported in 17 publications (n = 1338). After this review, six studies reporting on complications following unrestrictive MRgFUS were published. 4 retrospective cohorts (n = 372, 16, 71 and 33) and 2 prospective cohorts (n = 72 and 43).[17–22] Pooled complication rate of all these publications was 11.0% (213/1945), of which 99.1% (211/213)

were minor and 0.9% (2/213) were major. In conclusion, major complications are extremely rare probably due to the noninvasive nature of MRgFUS and temperature mapping and control during treatment.

Reintervention Rates

The systematic review by Verpalen and colleagues[15] is the only review reporting on reintervention rates after unrestrictive MRgFUS. They reported a range of pooled reintervention rates of 0% to 21% after 3 to 33.6 months follow-up. One additional unrestrictive MRgFUS study (retrospective cohort, n = 44) was published, with reintervention rates of 18.2% (8/44) (mean follow-up 40.0 ± 22.1 months).[23]

Reproductive Outcomes

Apart from myomectomy, MRgFUS is the only (noninvasive to minimally) invasive treatment for UFs that can be safely performed in women who still want to become pregnant. A systematic review by Anneveldt and colleagues[24] included 14 publications with 124 pregnancies, showing that pregnancy was safely possible after MRgFUS with pooled pregnancy rates of 36% (302/838), pooled live birth rates of 73% (69/94), and pooled miscarriage rates of 29.1% (25/86), without severe complications during delivery.

Comparative Studies

There is currently 1 systematic review published that reviews all studies that compare the results of MRgFUS treatment of UFs directly with those after UAE.[25] This systematic review included 4 comparative studies, all performing restrictive

MRgFUS. One of these studies, the FIRSTT trial, concerns a randomized controlled trial (RCT) paralleled by an observational cohort. The RCT included 27 patients in the MRgFUS group (mean NPV% 50.8 ± 22.2%) and 22 patients in the UAE group; the observational cohort consisted of 16 patients in the MRgFUS group (mean NPV% 46.1 ± 24.8%) and 18 patients in the UAE group. The FIRSTT trial showed a significantly greater improvement in tSSS and HRQoL in the UAE groups at 6, 12, and 24 months in comparison to the MRgFUS groups. However, UAE had longer recovery times (median 8 vs 4 days [P < .01]) and more analgesic use during recovery (P < .01). Reintervention rates of the RCT and observational cohort combined were 30.0% in the MRgFUS group (n = 43) and 12.5% in the UAE group (n = 40) (P = .064).[26,27] The other 3 included studies were retrospective cohort studies, including 51, 36, and 50 patients, with median NPV% of 38%, 36.4%, and 42.2%, respectively.[28–30] These retrospective cohort studies showed larger improvements in tSSS and HRQoL and lower reintervention rates in the UAE groups. However, it is important to keep in mind that part of the lower effectiveness of MRgFUS compared to UAE in these 4 studies can (at least partly) be explained by the rather low NPV% achieved due to the restrictive protocol used.

A prospective cohort study compared MRgFUS (restrictive protocol (NPV% not reported); n = 109) with abdominal hysterectomy (n = 83). The hysterectomy group showed greater improvement on tSSS and HRQoL, but there were significantly fewer major complications in the MRgFUS group (12.8% [14/109] vs. 36.4% in the surgery group [33/83] [P < .01]). In addition, the MRgFUS group reported return to work after 1.2 days and return to usual activities 2.7 days versus 19.2 and 17.4 days in the surgery group (P < .01).[31]

A retrospective cohort study comparing MRgFUS (unknown treatment protocol, NPV% not reported) (n = 68) to laparoscopic myomectomy (n = 64) showed no significant differences in HRQoL with median follow-up of 36.5 (24.2–41.7) and 31 (17.0–51.2) months, respectively (P = .62). Complication rates were not reported in this study.[32]

Costs and Reimbursement

Several cost-effectiveness studies are published, all showing that MRgFUS can be cost-effective compared to standard care.[33–37] However, all but 1 of these studies were published before 2015, when the long-term effects of MRgFUS were still uncertain and often restrictive MRgFUS was used, making these studies not directly applicable to current standard practice. A thorough cost-effectiveness analysis should be based on long-term results from controlled comparative trials, for example, the ongoing MYCHOICE trial in the Netherlands.[38] There is not yet widespread reimbursement for MRgFUS for UFs.

UTERINE ADENOMYOSIS

UA is the presence of endometrial-like tissue within the myometrial wall. Incidence is 1.0%, but UA is thought to be underdiagnosed.[39] Women with UA present mainly with menorrhagia (50%–60%) and dysmenorrhea (20%–80%), but chronic pelvic pain or infertility may also occur.[40] Conservative treatment consists of analgesics and hormonal therapy, with levonorgestrel-containing intrauterine devices proving most effective. However, conservative treatment is often insufficient and not suitable for women who want to conceive. The next treatment steps are UAE and, in selected cases, surgical removal of the adenomyosis spots or hysterectomy. Twenty-five percent of women with UA require hysterectomy to relieve symptoms.[41] The first MRgFUS treatment for UA was performed in 2006.[42] MRgFUS may be particularly beneficial for women who have failed conservative treatment, who wish to preserve fertility, or who prefer minimally invasive interventions.

Screening

MRgFUS eligibility in UA has the same anatomic eligibility criteria as UF, and a screening MRI is also required, as the presence of hyperintense spots in the UA lesion, abdominal wall thickness, and contrast enhancement on T1-weighted MRI negatively affect NPV%, while higher NPV% is associated with better clinical outcomes.[43,44] (Fig. 3) Kociuba and colleagues[45] investigated dynamic contrast enhancement of UA and showed that lower time-SI curves on dynamic contrast-enhanced T1-weighted MRI of UA compared to myometrium resulted in significantly higher NPV% than higher time-SI curves (89.2 ± 6.7% vs 42.4 ± 19.0% respectively [P < .01]).

Volume and Symptom Reduction

Cheung and colleagues[46] conducted the only systematic review available on treatment outcomes (5 publications, n = 84). Treatment outcomes were measured as reduction in UA lesion volume, reduction in tSSS, and reduction in pain scores. In order to provide as complete an overview as possible, we combined the results of this review with results of 3 other cohort studies, that is, the retrospective cohort

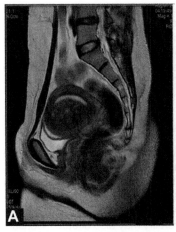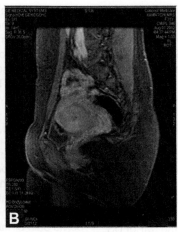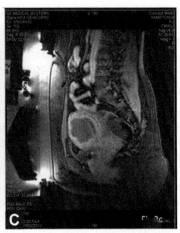

Fig. 3. MRI of uterine adenomyosis (UA) of the ventral uterine wall before and magnetic resonance–guided focused ultrasound surgery (MRgFUS). (*A*) Sagittal T2-weighted MRI of UA before MRgFUS. (*B*) Sagittal T1-weighted contrast MRI of UA before MRgFUS. (*C*) Sagittal T1-weighted contrast MRI of UA after MRgFUS showing non-perfused volume (NPV).[47] (Dev, B., Gadddam, S., Kumar, M., & Varadarajan, S. (2019). MR-guided focused ultrasound surgery: A novel non-invasive technique in the treatment of adenomyosis –18 month's follow-up of 12 cases. Indian Journal of Radiology and Imaging - New Series/Indian Journal of Radiology and Imaging/Indian Journal of Radiology & Imaging, 29(03), 284–288. https://doi.org/10.4103/ijri.ijri_53_19.)

studies by Jayaram and colleagues (n = 26)[18] and Huang and colleagues (n = 14),[47] and the prospective cohort study by Dev and colleagues (n = 12).[48] Range of mean UA lesion volume reductions were 28.3% to 34.6%, 2.0% to 54.0%, and 9.0% to 44.0% at 3, 6, and 12 months after MRgFUS, respectively.[18,46] Mean reductions in tSSS were 12.5% to 53.5%, 16.4% to 47.4%, 22.9% to 66.4%, and 54.4% at 3, 6, 12, and 18 months after MRgFUS, respectively.[46–48] Pain score reductions were 23.3% to 46.7%, 23.3% to 44.7%, and 27.6% to 66.7% at 3, 6, and 12 months after MRgFUS, respectively.[46–48]

Complications

All except Jayaram and colleagues reported on complications.[18,46,47] Pooled complication rate was 10.9% (12/110). The most common complication was prolonged buttock pain (4.5% [5/110]). There were 2 skin burns (1.8%) and no major complications.

Reintervention Rates

Two retrospective cohort studies reported reintervention rates 12 months after MRgFUS of 0% (0/26) and 14.3% (2/14).[18,48]

Reproductive Outcomes

Seven pregnancies after MRgFUS for UA have been described in 1 case report and 3 cohort studies (2 retrospective, 1 prospective; n = 53).[18,42,47,48] Two patients conceived following fertility treatment, 2

spontaneously. The mode of conception was not described in 3 patients. Five pregnancies resulted in live births and 2 pregnancies were ongoing. No obstetric complications were reported. These results suggest that pregnancy after MRgFUS for UA is safely possible.

Comparative Studies

There are no studies comparing MRgFUS with UAE, adenectomy, or hysterectomy for UA.

Costs

There are no studies investigating cost-effectiveness of MRgFUS for UA. There is no widespread reimbursement for MRgFUS for UA.

ABDOMINAL WALL ENDOMETRIOSIS

AWE occurs in 0.03% to 0.45% of women after gynecologic surgery, particularly cesarean sections. In AWE, endometrium-like cells are present in the abdominal wall and present as a cyclically painful, palpable nodule. Pharmacologic treatment with analgesics and hormonal therapy is often inadequate. In most cases, wide surgical excision is performed.[49] Since 2007, AWE is treated with FUS, mostly ultrasound guided (USgFUS).[50] Two case reports of MRgFUS for AWE have been published (n = 3).[51,52] No complications occurred; the AWE lesion volume decreased and pain complaints were significantly reduced in all patients (**Fig. 4**).

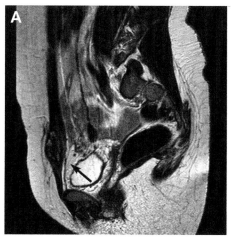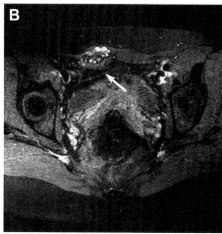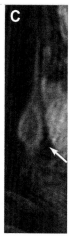

Fig. 4. (*A*) Sagittal T2-weighted MRI showing abdominal wall endometriosis lesion of 38 × 23 × 39 mm in right rectus abdominis muscle (*black arrow*). (*B*) Axial T1-weighted MRI with fat suppression showing areas with high T1 signal indicating the presence of blood products (*white arrow*). (*C*) Sagittal T1-weighted MRI post-gadolinium immediately after magnetic resonance–guided focused ultrasound surgery (MRgFUS), showing non-perfused volume of greater than 50% (*white arrow*).[52] (Bertine L. Stehouwer et al., Magnetic Resonance Imaging–Guided High-Intensity Focused Ultrasound is a Noninvasive Treatment Modality for Patients with Abdominal Wall Endometriosis, Journal of Minimally Invasive Gynecology, 25 (7), 2018, 1300-1304, https://doi.org/10.1016/j.jmig.2018.03.018.)

PALLIATIVE TREATMENT OF RECURRENT GYNECOLOGIC MALIGNANCY

To date, there is only 1 publication on PRGMs. Imseeh and colleagues (2021)[53] palliatively treated 11 PRGMs with MRgFUS in 10 patients who were ineligible for any other therapy (**Fig. 5**). Five patients responded to therapy. Responders had lower worst pain scores than non-responders up to the 90 days follow-up. Although physical function did not improve in the participants, emotional function did, as assessed by the Brief Pain Inventory short form, 15-item European Organization for the Research and Treatment of Cancer Quality of Life Questionnaire For Palliative Care, and European Quality of Life 5 Dimensions 5 Level Version. Two patients experienced skin burns (grade one n = 1; grade two n = 1). No other complications occurred.

This publication shows that MRgFUS may be considered in the palliative treatment of PRGMs, but more research is needed to conclude on the efficacy and safety of MRgFUS for this indication.

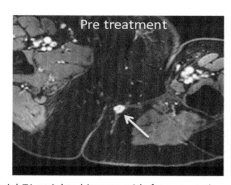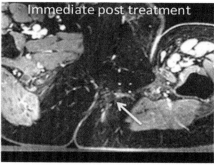

Fig. 5. Axial T1-weighted images with fat suppression pulse and after contrast enhancement with gadolinium chelate before and after magnetic resonance–guided focused ultrasound surgery (MRgFUS) of an extra-pelvic tumor. The pretreatment image shows the enhancing nodule of recurrent tumor in the left ischio-rectal fat (*yellow arrow*). Immediately post-treatment there is complete ablation of this enhancing lesion (*yellow arrow*).[53] (Imseeh, G. et al., (2021). Feasibility of palliating recurrent gynecological tumors with MRGHIFU: comparison of symptom, quality-of-life, and imaging response in intra and extra-pelvic disease. International Journal of Hyperthermia, 38(1), 623–632. https://doi.org/10.1080/02656736.2021.1904154.)

DISCUSSION

This review on MRgFUS for gynecologic indications shows that there is a relatively large body of evidence that MRgFUS is an effective and safe treatment for UF and UA. For AWE and PRGMs, MRgFUS treatment shows promise in relieving pain symptoms, but more research is needed. Overall, large comparative trials are rare. Where larger multicenter trials exist, they involve relatively small numbers of patients.

Reimbursement

There is no widespread reimbursement for MRgFUS for any of the gynecologic indications. In today's health care landscape of rising medical costs and increasing responsibility of health care providers to reduce these costs, it is important to assess both the (long-term) effectiveness and cost-effectiveness of a new treatment compared to standard care in order to qualify for reimbursement. However, the strong preference that women may have for 1 treatment over another, may make it very difficult to conduct comparative trials.[26] For example, women with UFs or UA younger than 40 years often prefer treatments that ensure fertility preservation and low complication rates but sufficient symptom relief.[54] While hysterectomy relieves symptoms, it is not compatible with fertility preservation and there is an increased risk of complications and generally long recovery times. Hysterectomy can also have a major emotional impact, as the uterus symbolizes femininity and fertility.[55] UAE carries a risk of premature ovarian failure affecting the ability to have children and surgical myomectomy carries risk of surgical complications.[56,57] In theory, MRgFUS for UFs and UA may be particularly beneficial for (younger) women who wish to conceive and for perimenopausal/postmenopausal women because they have a reduced risk of recurrence of the UF or UA. Currently, studies inventorying patient preference are lacking.

There are also other barriers to conducting controlled prospective trials and RCTs such as funding, time, and the large sample sizes needed. Therefore, consortia should be established to conduct these studies and make progress toward reimbursement of MRgFUS for gynecologic indications. Furthermore, support from (international) radiological and gynecologic societies will raise awareness and may help to establish and support such consortia.

Implementation in Clinical Practice

Reimbursement is only the first step in clinical adoption of MRgFUS in gynecology. To understand the difficulties in implementation, the following paradox must be addressed: UFs and UA are common conditions, that almost all gynecologists see frequently, but for noninvasive treatments such as MRgFUS, patients have to be referred to a center of expertise. This means that gynecologists need to counsel for treatments they may not be familiar with. To overcome this barrier, structured referral pathways should be implemented, counseling information should be easily accessible to both gynecologists and patients, and participation in hybrid multicenter multidisciplinary consultations should be offered to referring gynecologists.[58] Closed loop feedback should be provided to the referring clinicians to increase their familiarity with the MRgFUS treatment and its outcomes and their willingness to provide counseling for noninvasive treatments.

Possibilities of Magnetic Resonance–Guided Focused Ultrasound Surgery Within Gynecology

We have focused on MRgFUS for gynecologic indications in this review, but it is important to note that several additional gynecologic indications, for example, deep infiltrating endometriosis and cesarean scar pregnancies, have been treated with USgFUS.[59,60] Theoretically, these indications are also eligible for MRgFUS. MRgFUS with real-time MRI visualization, anatomic planning, and thermal mapping may even be superior for some indications, possibly leading to higher NPV% and therefore better clinical outcomes and fewer recurrences.[61] On the other hand, USgFUS is more convenient, and costs are lower compared to MRgFUS. Therefore, USgFUS may be easier to implement locally. Comparative studies of MRgFUS versus USgFUS in gynecologic indications should be conducted.

SUMMARY

MRgFUS is promising as an effective and safe treatment for UFs, UA, AWE, and PRGMs, but controlled prospective cohort studies or RCTs with a high LoE on long-term (cost)effectiveness, which are needed for reimbursement and subsequent clinical adoption of the technique, are still lacking (Appendix 2 – Research agenda).

CLINICS CARE POINTS

- In gynaecology, MRgFUS has been studied and used primarily for the treatment of uterine fibroids and adenomyosis. MRgFUS treatment for these indications results in a reduction in the volume of the targeted lesion, leading to a reduction in symptoms and an improvement in health-related quality of life. Both indications have low complication rates, with major complications being particularly rare. However, there is still a lack of research on long-term re-intervention rates, reproductive outcomes, cost-effectiveness and how MRgFUS compares with standard care for both indications.

- MRgFUS treatment of abdominal wall endometriosis (AWE) and palliative treatment of recurrent gynaecological malignancies has been described in a small number of patients, showing promising results in reducing pain symptoms without major complications for both indications. However, research is still at an early stage.

DISCLOSURE

The authors have nothing to disclose.

REFERENCES

1. Siedek F, Yeo SY, Heijman E, et al. Magnetic resonance-guided high-intensity focused ultrasound (MR-HIFU): technical background and overview of current clinical applications (Part 1). RöFo - Fortschritte auf dem Gebiet der Röntgenstrahlen und der bildgebenden Verfahren 2019; 191(06):522–30.
2. Borah BJ, Nicholson WK, Bradley L, et al. The impact of uterine leiomyomas: a national survey of affected women. Am J Obstet Gynecol 2013;209: 4319.e20.
3. Howick J., Chalmers I., Glasziou P., et al., The Oxford Levels of Evidence 2. Oxford Centre for Evidence-Based Medicine. Available at: https://www.cebm.ox.ac.uk/resources/levels-of-evidence/ocebm-levels-of-evidence. (Accessed 21 November, 2023).
4. Schünemann H, Brozek J, Guyatt G, et al. GRADE Handbook. GRADE Handbook. 2013. Available at: https://gdt.gradepro.org/app/handbook/handbook.html. [Accessed 21 November 2023].
5. Stewart E, Cookson C, Gandolfo R, et al. Epidemiology of uterine fibroids: a systematic review. BJOG 2017;124(10):1501–12.
6. Rueff L, Raman S. Clinical and technical aspects of MR-guided high intensity focused ultrasound for treatment of symptomatic uterine fibroids. Semin Intervent Radiol 2013;30(04):347–53.
7. Duc NM, Keserci B. Review of influential clinical factors in reducing the risk of unsuccessful MRI-guided HIFU treatment outcome of uterine fibroids. Diagn Interventional Radiol 2018;24(5): 283–91.
8. Verpalen IM, Veer-ten Kate M, de Boer E, et al. Development and clinical evaluation of a 3-step modified manipulation protocol for MRI-guided high-intensity focused ultrasound of uterine fibroids. Eur Radiol 2020;30(7):3869–78.
9. Funaki K, Fukunishi H, Funaki T, et al. Magnetic resonance-guided focused ultrasound surgery for uterine fibroids: relationship between the therapeutic effects and signal intensity of preexisting T2-weighted magnetic resonance images. Am J Obstet Gynecol 2007;196(2):184.e1–6.
10. Jiang L, Yu JW, Yang MJ, et al. Ultrasound-guided HIFU for uterine fibroids of hyperintense on T2-weighted MR imaging with or without GnRH-analogue-pretreated: A propensity score matched cohort study. Front Surg 2022;9. https://doi.org/10.3389/fsurg.2022.975839.
11. Verpalen IM, Anneveldt KJ, Vos PC, et al. Use of multiparametric MRI to characterize uterine fibroid tissue types. Magnetic Resonance Materials in Physics, Biology and Medicine 2020;33(5): 689–700.
12. Keserci B, Duc NM. Magnetic resonance imaging parameters in predicting the treatment outcome of high-intensity focused ultrasound ablation of uterine fibroids with an immediate nonperfused volume ratio of at least 90. Acad Radiol 2018;25(10):1257–69.
13. Bitton RR, Fast A, Vu KN, et al. What predicts durable symptom relief of uterine fibroids treated with MRI-guided focused ultrasound? A multicenter trial in 8 academic centers. Eur Radiol 2023;33(11): 7360–70.
14. Slotman DJ, Nijholt IM, Schutte JM, et al. No incision required for long-lasting symptom relief in a selection of women suffering from uterine fibroids. Eur Radiol 2023;33(11):7357–9.
15. Verpalen IM, Anneveldt KJ, Nijholt IM, et al. Magnetic resonance-high intensity focused ultrasound (MR-HIFU) therapy of symptomatic uterine fibroids with unrestrictive treatment protocols: a systematic review and meta-analysis. Eur J Radiol 2019;120: 108700.
16. Lozinski T, Filipowska J, Pyka M, et al. Magnetic resonance-guided high-intensity ultrasound (MR-HIFU) in the treatment of symptomatic uterine fibroids — five-year experience. Ginekol Pol 2022; 93(3):185–94.
17. Wang Y, Wang ZB, Xu YH. Efficacy, efficiency, and safety of magnetic resonance-guided high-intensity focused ultrasound for ablation of uterine fibroids: comparison with ultrasound-guided method. Korean J Radiol 2018;19(4):724.
18. Huang Y, Zhou S, Wang J, et al. Efficacy and safety of magnetic resonance-guided focused ultrasound surgery (MRgFUS) ablation in the management of abnormal uterine bleeding due to uterine leiomyoma or adenomyosis. Am J Transl Res 2022;14(1):656–63.

19. Keserci B, Duc NM, Nadarajan C, et al. Volumetric MRI-guided, high-intensity focused ultrasound ablation of uterine leiomyomas: ASEAN preliminary experience. Diagn Interventional Radiol 2020;26(3):207–15.

20. Kociuba J, Łoziński T, Zgliczyńska M, et al. Occurrence of adverse events after magnetic resonance-guided high-intensity focused ultrasound (MR-HIFU) therapy in symptomatic uterine fibroids—a retrospective case-control study. Int J Hyperther 2023;40(1). https://doi.org/10.1080/02656736.2023.2219436.

21. Inbar Y, Machtinger R, Barnett-Itzhaki Z, et al. MRI guided focused ultrasound (MRgFUS) treatment for uterine fibroids among women with and without abdominal scars. Int J Hyperther 2021;38(1):1672–6.

22. Browne JE, Gorny KR, Hangiandreou NJ, et al. Comparison of clinical performance between two generations of magnetic resonance-guided focused ultrasound systems in treatments of uterine leiomyomas. Acad Radiol 2021;28(10):1361–7.

23. Verpalen IM, de Boer JP, Linstra M, et al. The Focused Ultrasound Myoma Outcome Study (FU-MOS); a retrospective cohort study on long-term outcomes of MR-HIFU therapy. Eur Radiol 2020; 30(5):2473–82.

24. Anneveldt KJ, van 't Oever HJ, Nijholt IM, et al. Systematic review of reproductive outcomes after high intensity focused ultrasound treatment of uterine fibroids. Eur J Radiol 2021;141:109801.

25. Jeng CJ, Long CY, Chuang LT. Comparison of magnetic resonance-guided high-intensity focused ultrasound with uterine artery embolization for the treatment of uterine myoma: a systematic literature review and meta-analysis. Taiwan J Obstet Gynecol 2020;59(5):691–7.

26. Laughlin-Tommaso S, Barnard EP, AbdElmagied AM, et al. FIRSTT study: randomized controlled trial of uterine artery embolization vs focused ultrasound surgery. Am J Obstet Gynecol 2019;220(2):174.e1–13.

27. Barnard EP, AbdElmagied AM, Vaughan LE, et al. Periprocedural outcomes comparing fibroid embolization and focused ultrasound: a randomized controlled trial and comprehensive cohort analysis. Am J Obstet Gynecol 2017;216(5):500.e11.

28. Froeling V, Meckelburg K, Scheurig-Muenkler C, et al. Midterm results after uterine artery embolization versus MR-guided high-intensity focused ultrasound treatment for symptomatic uterine fibroids. Cardiovasc Intervent Radiol 2013;36(6):1508–13.

29. Froeling V, Meckelburg K, Schreiter NF, et al. Outcome of uterine artery embolization versus MR-guided high-intensity focused ultrasound treatment for uterine fibroids: Long-term results. Eur J Radiol 2013;82(12):2265–9.

30. Ikink ME, Nijenhuis RJ, Verkooijen HM, et al. Volumetric MR-guided high-intensity focused ultrasound versus uterine artery embolisation for treatment of symptomatic uterine fibroids: comparison of symptom improvement and reintervention rates. Eur Radiol 2014;24(10):2649–57.

31. Taran FA, Tempany CMC, Regan L, et al. Magnetic resonance-guided focused ultrasound (MRgFUS) compared with abdominal hysterectomy for treatment of uterine leiomyomas. Ultrasound Obstet Gynecol 2009;34(5):572–8.

32. Mohr-Sasson A, Machtinger R, Mashiach R, et al. Long-term outcome of MR-guided focused ultrasound treatment and laparoscopic myomectomy for symptomatic uterine fibroid tumors. Am J Obstet Gynecol 2018;219(4):375. e1-.e7.

33. Cain-Nielsen AH, Moriarty JP, Stewart EA, et al. Cost–effectiveness of uterine-preserving procedures for the treatment of uterine fibroid symptoms in the USA. J Comp Eff Res 2014;3(5):503–14.

34. Kong CY, Meng L, Omer ZB, et al. MRI-guided focused ultrasound surgery for uterine fibroid treatment: a cost-effectiveness analysis. Am J Roentgenol 2014;203(2):361–71.

35. Borah BJ, Carls GS, Moore BJ, et al. Cost comparison between uterine-sparing fibroid treatments one year following treatment. J Ther Ultrasound 2014;2(1):7.

36. Babashov V, Palimaka S, Blackhouse G, et al. Magnetic resonance-guided high-intensity focused ultrasound (MRgHIFU) for treatment of symptomatic uterine fibroids: an economic analysis. Ont Health Technol Assess Ser 2015;15(5):1–61.

37. Ferrario L, Garagiola E, Gerardi C, et al. Innovative and conventional "conservative" technologies for the treatment of uterine fibroids in Italy: a multidimensional assessment. Health Econ Rev 2022;12(1):21.

38. Anneveldt KJ, Nijholt IM, Schutte JM, et al. Comparison of (cost-)effectiveness of magnetic resonance image–guided high-intensity–focused ultrasound with standard (minimally) invasive fibroid treatments: protocol for a multicenter randomized controlled trial (MYCHOICE). JMIR Res Protoc 2021;10(11):e29467.

39. Upson K, Missmer SA. Epidemiology of Adenomyosis. Semin Reprod Med 2020;38(02/03):089–107.

40. Li X, Liu X, Guo S. Clinical profiles of 710 premenopausal women with adenomyosis who underwent hysterectomy. J Obstet Gynaecol Res 2014;40(2):485–94.

41. Cope AG, Ainsworth AJ, Stewart EA. Current and future medical therapies for adenomyosis. Semin Reprod Med 2020;38(02/03):151–6.

42. Rabinovici J, Inbar Y, Eylon SC, et al. Pregnancy and live birth after focused ultrasound surgery for symptomatic focal adenomyosis: a case report. Hum Reprod 2006;21(5):1255–9.

43. Gong C, Setzen R, Liu Z, et al. High intensity focused ultrasound treatment of adenomyosis: The relationship between the features of magnetic resonance imaging on T2 weighted images and the therapeutic efficacy. Eur J Radiol 2017;89:117–22.

44. Zhang L, Rao F, Setzen R. High intensity focused ultrasound for the treatment of adenomyosis: selection criteria, efficacy, safety and fertility. Acta Obstet Gynecol Scand 2017;96(6):707–14.

45. Keserci B, Duc NM. The role of T1 perfusion-based classification in predicting the outcome of magnetic resonance-guided high-intensity focused ultrasound treatment of adenomyosis. Int J Hyperther 2018; 34(3):306–14.

46. Cheung VYT. Current status of high-intensity focused ultrasound for the management of uterine adenomyosis. Ultrasonography 2017;36(2):95–102.

47. Dev B, Gadddam S, Kumar M, et al. MR-guided focused ultrasound surgery: A novel non-invasive technique in the treatment of adenomyosis –18 month's follow-up of 12 cases. Indian J Radiol Imag 2019; 29(03):284–8.

48. Jayaram R, Subbarayan K, Mithraprabhu S, et al. Heavy menstrual bleeding and dysmenorrhea are improved by magnetic resonance guided focused ultrasound surgery (MRgFUS) of adenomyosis. Fertil Res Pract 2016;2(1):8.

49. Benedetto C, Cacozza D, de Sousa Costa D, et al. Abdominal wall endometriosis: Report of 83 cases. Int J Gynecol Obstet 2022;159(2):530–6.

50. Wang Y, Wang W, Wang L, et al. Ultrasound-guided high-intensity focused ultrasound treatment for abdominal wall endometriosis: Preliminary results. Eur J Radiol 2011;79(1):56–9.

51. Nguyen M. Magnetic resonance imaging-guided high-intensity focused ultrasound ablation for endometriosis of the abdominal wall. Gynecol Minim Invasive Ther 2020;9(1):45.

52. Stehouwer BL, Braat MNG, Veersema S. Magnetic resonance imaging–guided high-intensity focused ultrasound is a noninvasive treatment modality for patients with abdominal wall endometriosis. J Minim Invasive Gynecol 2018;25(7):1300–4.

53. Imseeh G, Giles SL, Taylor A, et al. Feasibility of palliating recurrent gynecological tumors with MRGHIFU: comparison of symptom, quality-of-life, and imaging response in intra and extra-pelvic disease. Int J Hyperther 2021;38(1):623–32.

54. Babalola O, Gebben D, Tarver ME, et al. Patient Preferences Regarding Surgical Treatment Methods for Symptomatic Uterine Fibroids. Ther Innov Regul Sci 2023;57(5):976–86.

55. Li N, Shen C, Wang R, et al. The real experience with women's hysterectomy: A meta-synthesis of qualitative research evidence. Nurs Open 2023;10(2): 435–49.

56. Czuczwar P, Stepniak A, Wrona W, et al. The influence of uterine artery embolisation on ovarian reserve, fertility, and pregnancy outcomes – a review of literature. Menopausal Review 2016;4:205–9.

57. Tanos V, Berry KE, Frist M, et al. Prevention and Management of Complications in Laparoscopic Myomectomy. BioMed Res Int 2018;2018:1–9.

58. Papoutsi C, Boaden R, Foy R, et al. Challenges for implementation science. In: Raine R, Fitzpatrick R, Barratt H, et al, editors. Challenges, solutions and future directions in the evaluation of service innovations in health care and public health. Health Serv Deliv Res; 2016. p. 121–32.

59. Liu Y, Wang L, Zhu X. Efficacy and Safety of High-intensity Focused Ultrasound Compared with Uterine Artery Embolization in Cesarean Section Pregnancy: A Meta-analysis. J Minim Invasive Gynecol 2023;30(6):446–54.

60. Philip C, Warembourg S, Dairien M, et al. Transrectal high-intensity focused ultrasound (HIFU) for management of rectosigmoid deep infiltrating endometriosis: results of Phase-I clinical trial. Ultrasound Obstet Gynecol 2020;56(3):431–42.

61. Edwards K, Tsai S, Kothari A. Clinical and imaging features of abdominal wall endometriomas. Australas J Ultrasound Med 2018;21(1):24–8.

APPENDIX 1: LEVEL OF EVIDENCE (LoE) AND GRADE OF RECOMMENDATION (GoR) EXPLAINED AND PROVIDED PER INDICATION

Table 1
Level of evidence (Oxford Center of Evidence-Based Medicine 2011) and grade of recommendation

Level of Evidence

Question	Level 1[a]	Level 2[a]	Level 3[a]	Level 4[a]	Level 5[a]
How common is the problem?	Local and current random sample surveys (or censuses)	Systematic review of surveys that allow matching to local circumstances[b]	Local non-random sample[b]	Case series[b]	n/a
Is this diagnostic or monitoring test accurate? (Diagnosis)	Systematic review of cross-sectional studies with consistently applied reference standard and blinding	Individual cross-sectional studies with consistently applied reference standard and blinding	Non-consecutive studies, or studies without consistently applied reference standards[b]	Case-control studies, or "poor or non-independent" reference standard[b]	Mechanism-based reasoning
What will happen if we do not add a therapy? (Prognosis)	Systematic review of inception cohort studies	Inception cohort studies	Cohort study or control arm of randomized trial[a]	Case series or case-control studies, or poor-quality prognostic cohort study[b]	n/a
Does this intervention help? (Treatment benefits)	Systematic review of randomized trials or n-of-1 trials	Randomized trial or observational study with dramatic effect	Non-randomized controlled cohort/follow-up study[b]	Case series, case-control, or historically controlled studies[b]	Mechanism-based reasoning
What are the common harms? (Treatment harms)	Systematic review of randomized trials, systematic review of nested case-control studies, n-of-1 trial with the patient you are raising the question about, or observational study with dramatic effect	Individual randomized trial or (exceptionally) observational study with dramatic effect	Non-randomized controlled cohort/follow-up study (post-marketing surveillance) provided there are sufficient numbers to rule out a common harm. (For long-term harms the duration of follow-up must be sufficient.)[b]		Mechanism-based reasoning
What are the rare harms? (Treatment Harms)	Systematic review of randomized trials or n-of-1 trial	Randomized trial or (exceptionally) observational study with dramatic effect			

Is this (early detection) test worthwhile? (Screening)	Systematic review of randomized trials	Randomized trial	Non-randomized controlled cohort/follow-up study[b]	Case series, case-control, or historically controlled studies[b]	Mechanism-based reasoning
GoR	A	B	C	D	n/a
Descriptor	Strong recommendation (Consistent LoE 1 studies)	Recommendation (Consistent LoE 2 or 3 studies or extrapolations from LoE 1 studies)	Suggestion (LoE 4 studies or extrapolations from LoE 2 or 3 studies)	Suggestion (LoE 5 evidence or troublingly inconsistent or inconclusive studies of any level)	n/a

Abbreviations: GoR, grade of recommendation; LoE, level of evidence.

[a] Level may be graded down on the basis of study quality, imprecision, indirectness (study PICO does not match questions PICO) because of inconsistency between studies, or because the absolute effect size is very small; Level may be graded up if there is a large or very large effect size.

[b] As always, a systematic review is generally better than an individual study.

Table 2
Level of evidence and grade of recommendation per indication per outcome

Indication Outcomes	Uterine Fibroids		Adenomyosis		Abdominal wall endometriosis		Recurrent Gynecologic Malignancies	
	LoE	GoR	LoE	GoR	LoE	GoR	LoE	GoR
Screening methods	2	B	3	C	4	C	4	C
Volume and symptom reduction	2	B	2	B	4	C	4	C
Common complications	2	B	2	B	4	C	4	C
Rare complications	2	B	3	C	4	D	4	D
Reintervention rates	2	B	3	C	LOD	LOD	LOD	LOD
Reproductive outcomes	3	C	4	C	n.a.	n.a.	n.a.	n.a.
Comparison to other treatments	2	B	LOD	LOD	LOD	LOD	LOD	LOD

Abbreviations: GoR, grade of recommendation; LOD, lack of data; LoE, level of evidence; n.a., not applicable.

APPENDIX 2: RESEARCH AGENDA

- Controlled prospective trial or RCT in patients with uterine fibroids who are actively trying to conceive, comparing expectant management, myomectomy and MRgFUS, with time to conception and miscarriage rates as primary outcomes.
- Controlled prospective trial or RCT including patients with symptomatic uterine adenomyosis, comparing pharmacologic treatment with surgical treatment, UAE and MRgFUS, with tSSS, HRQoL, recurrence rates, reintervention rates, and costs as primary outcomes.
- Controlled prospective trial or RCT including patients with symptomatic abdominal wall endometriosis, comparing MRgFUS with surgery, with symptom reduction, reintervention rates, and costs as primary outcomes.
- Patient preference studies for the treatment of benign gynecological pathologies (eg, uterine fibroids and adenomyosis), including pharmacologic, noninvasive, minimally invasive, and surgical interventions.
- Comparison of USgFUS with MRgFUS for long-term effectivity and safety in gynecologic indications.
- Research on expanding MRgFUS indications within gynecology.

MR-guided Focused Ultrasound Focal Therapy for Prostate Cancer

Vanessa Murad, MD[a], Nathan Perlis, MD, MSc, FRCSC[b], Sangeet Ghai, MD[a],*

KEYWORDS

- Prostate cancer • MR imaging • MR imaging-guided focused ultrasound

KEY POINTS

- Patient selection is crucial for focal therapy (FT) success. FT may be considered for patients with intermediate risk, localized, image distinct, biopsy-confirmed prostate cancer.
- The main advantages of MR imaging-guided focused ultrasound (MRgFUS) FT include the more accurate localization of the lesion in 3 planes and the real-time thermal monitoring during treatment.
- MRgFUS represents a widely studied, feasible and safe technique, with good clinical and oncological results.

INTRODUCTION

Prostate cancer (PCa) is one of the leading cancers diagnosed in men in most Western countries. The extent of the disease at the time of diagnosis determines the treatment and impacts the morbidity and mortality. Risk stratification is determined by tumor, node, metastasis classification system (TNM) staging, Gleason Grade Group (GG; **Table 1**), and prostate-specific antigen (PSA) levels.[1] The management of localized disease has evolved significantly in recent years, contributing to the decreasing mortality despite the increasing incidence. It is estimated that only 2.4% of diagnosed patients will die from this cause.[2,3] Focal therapy (FT), defined as the guided ablation of an image distinct and biopsy-confirmed cancerous lesion with a safety margin,[4,5] has emerged as a promising alternative to selectively treat areas of localized clinically significant (cs) PCa (GG ≥2) while preserving healthy prostatic tissue and minimizing the potential for treatment-related side effects of radical therapies including sexual and urinary

dysfunction.[6–9] FT may be considered for patients with intermediate-grade localized disease, with the aim of eradicating all clinically significant PCa (csPCa) foci, thus changing the natural course of disease and the patient's prognosis.[3–5,10] About 20% to 30% of PCas are unifocal and/or unilateral, which makes them suitable for FT.[11]

To date, there are no strict or universal eligibility criteria for FT[12] but is determined by multiple factors mainly GG, tumor volume, and life expectancy. However, multiple expert consensuses have been published in recent years including 2 international Delphi Consensus Projects,[5,13] the American Urological Association recommendations,[6] the Imperial College of London criteria,[14] and the University of California collaborative consensus statement[15]; the different eligibility recommendations are summarized in **Box 1**. In our experience, ideal candidates are those with MR imaging-visible lesions measuring up to 15 mm, clinical stage T1c to T2a, GG2 or GG3 disease, PSA level less than 15 to 20 ng/mL (depending upon gland size and PSA density), and life expectancy greater than 5 to

[a] Joint Department of Medical Imaging, University Health Network - Mount Sinai Hospital – Women's, College Hospital, University of Toronto, Toronto, Ontario, Canada; [b] Division of Urology, Department of Surgical Oncology, University Health Network, University of Toronto, Toronto, Ontario, Canada
* Corresponding author. 1PMB-292, Toronto General Hospital, 585 University Avenue, Toronto, Ontario M5G 2N2, Canada.
E-mail address: Sangeet.Ghai@uhn.ca

Magn Reson Imaging Clin N Am 32 (2024) 629–640
https://doi.org/10.1016/j.mric.2024.04.001
1064-9689/24/© 2024 Elsevier Inc. All rights reserved.

Table 1
Grade group and Gleason score classification for prostate cancer[49,50]

Grade Group	Gleason Score	Tumor Grade
1	≤ 6	Low
2	7 (3+4)	Intermediate
3	7 (4+3)	Intermediate
4	8	High
5	9–10	High

10 years.[1] General exclusion criteria include locally advanced or extraprostatic disease, multiple sites of clinically significant disease, no visible tumor on MR imaging, and any other contraindications for undergoing MR imaging[1] or template mapping biopsy. Other potential exclusion criteria may vary depending on the energy source used, that is, the presence of calcifications along the treatment path and visible tumor greater than 5 cm from the

Box 1
Summary of eligibility recommendations for focal therapy according to multiple expert consensuses: International Delphi Consensus Project,[42] Delphi Consensus Project,[13] American Urological Association[6]

Tumor grade

- Intermediate-grade PCa (GG2 and GG3)
- Low-grade PCa (GG1) when:
  o Lesion measuring greater than 6 mm on MR imaging[14]
  o High genomic risk[5,15]

Tumor volume

- Tumor foci less than 1.5 mL on mpMR imaging or involving less than 20% of the prostate[5]
- Tumor foci up to 3 mL or involving 25% if localized to one hemigland[5]

Life expectancy

- When overall expectancy (excluding PCa diagnosis) is greater than the expected disease-related mortality[14]

PSA (no consensus on cutoff value, not routinely considered for decision-making)

- Prebiopsy PSA less than 20 ng/mL[14,15]

Abbreviations: GG, Gleason Grade Group; mpMR imaging, multiparametric MR imaging; PCa, prostate cancer; PSA, prostate-specific antigen.

rectum may be contraindications for high-intensity focused ultrasound (HIFU)[16] while energy sources lacking a mechanism for rectal cooling or protection, may not be suited for ablation of midline posterior tumors in close proximity to the rectum.

FT can be directed to a defined focus (targeted ablation) or limited to a specific region (quadrant ablation or hemiablation). FT templates refer to the standardized nomenclature to define the anatomic boundaries of ablation, which may vary based on the specific type of energy source employed and the ablation guidance[17] (**Fig. 1**). There are different energy sources that can be used to destroy cancer cells as part of an FT strategy, among which HIFU has been the most extensively studied.[18] Other techniques include cryoablation,[19] photodynamic laser therapy,[20] transurethral ultrasound ablation (TULSA),[3] focal laser ablation,[21,22] and irreversible electroporation.[23]

HIFU ablation techniques are based on hyperthermia-induced tissue necrosis and can be administered under ultrasound (US) guidance or under MR imaging guidance, the latter demonstrating several advantages.[9,17,24] The first clinical use of focused US (FUS) for ablation therapy was introduced in China in the 1980s.[25] Currently, there are different approaches to MR imaging-guided HIFU/high-intensity directed ultrasound (HIDU) techniques, including transrectal MR imaging-guided FUS (MRgFUS) and TULSA. In the current article, we present a detailed review of the use of MRgFUS based on the most updated literature.

MR IMAGING GUIDANCE: ADVANTAGES AND LIMITATIONS

Multiparametric (mp) MR imaging continues being the main modality for the detection and follow-up of men with csPCa.[26] Since mpMR imaging is considered the standard of care for the detection of csPCa, more recent studies have focused on MR imaging-guided FT, showing excellent results. MR imaging-guided FT enables better localization and definition of the lesion in 3 planes for treatment planning, which in turn allows better targeting, and real-time thermal monitoring (MR-thermometry) permitting intraprocedural optimization of ablation temperatures and treatment margins.[3,27–29] These advantages translate into a targeted approach, enabling a smaller and precise ablation volume. Several studies have reported that smaller ablation volumes result in better functional outcomes highlighting the benefit of targeted ablation.[30] For instance, results of the phase II trial using MRgFUS by Ghai and colleagues[31] noted that participants with larger ablations (≥ 15 cc vs <15 cc) had significantly greater erectile dysfunction at 6 weeks

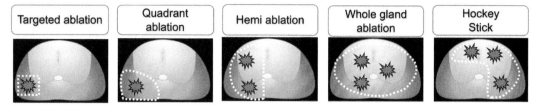

Fig. 1. Templates for focal therapy.

following treatment. It is, however, known that MR imaging underestimates the true extent of disease,[32–34] and therefore, targeted FT approach also requires adequate margins beyond the MR imaging-visible tumor. Treatment under MR imaging guidance allows precise inclusion of adequate margins in all planes for treatment planning.

MR imaging-guidance has certain limitations, specifically the need for MR-compatible devices for therapy and anesthesia, and longer procedure times, both leading to additional costs.[31]

MAGNETIC RESONANCE-GUIDED FOCUSED ULTRASOUND TECHNIQUE

This technique uses a specific endorectal probe (Food and Drug Administration [FDA]-approved device Exablate 2100; Insightec) capable of generating high-frequency US waves within the range 0.8 to 3.5 mHz to a target area, causing heating to attain raised temperatures of greater than 60°C in a few seconds, leading to coagulation necrosis (**Fig. 2**). The phased-array transducer is

composed of approximately 1000 elements, and its configuration enables the system to steer the US beam to the desired location in the prostate based on gland anatomy and tumor location on MR images.[35] The procedure is performed under general anesthesia or sedation with the patient in the lithotomy position on a modified MR imaging table. A Foley catheter is placed to facilitate continuous bladder drainage, and in cases where the urethra is included in the planned ablation volume, a suprapubic catheter may be necessary. The endorectal probe is placed within the rectum and filled with degassed water circulating at 14°C to ensure rectal cooling. Initial images are obtained to ensure that there are not air bubbles within the endorectal balloon along the treatment path. Air bubbles can disrupt the transmission of US waves and result in uneven or inadequate heating of the targeted prostatic tissue. Subsequently, T2-weighted (T2W) and diffusion-weighted (DW) images are acquired for planning and manual contouring of the prostate gland and of the tumor including margins of up to 10 mm when possible;

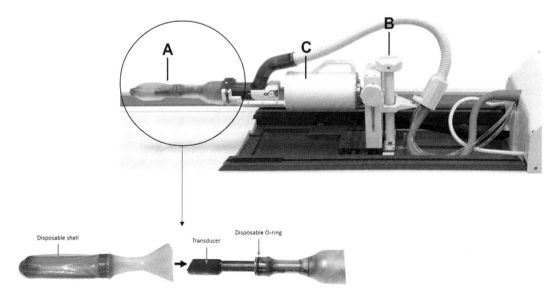

Fig. 2. FDA-approved endorectal probe device (Exablate 2100; Insightec). (A) The 990 elements phased-array transducer inside a single-use disposable shell. (B) Mechanical positioning unit, for fixing the probe in place during the procedure. (C) Robotic automatic motion unit.

contouring of the urethra, rectal wall, and neurovascular bundle are also performed. The software generates the specific treatment plan including the required energy level and number of sonications.[17,27,35,36] Once the planning is completed, initial subtherapeutic sonications are given for verification, followed by multiple consecutive treatment sonications, prioritizing the protection of sensitive structures such as the rectal wall, external urethral sphincter, and bladder wall.[27] Macrosonications containing multiple nominal sonication spots are delivered on each axial slice encompassing the contoured tumor and margins. It is important to consider that because the penetration of US waves is limited, the success rates may be decreased in patients with large prostatic volumes, anteriorly located lesions, and when calcifications are present in the treatment beam path.[3,16]

During the ablation process, real-time temperature feedback is provided through MR thermography, consisting in a noninvasive temperature mapping in the area being treated. This optimizes tumor ablative temperatures and prevents injury to the surrounding healthy tissues. There are several methods to measure temperature-related changes on MR imaging, of which the proton resonance frequency (PRF) shift of water protons is the most frequently used; other methods include T1 and T2 relaxation time of water protons, proton density, magnetization transfer, and diffusion coefficient.[16,18,21,37] PRF MR thermography is based on water hydrogen bonds disrupting at elevated temperatures, resulting in decreased chemical shift and decreased resonance frequency for water protons. The software creates maps in gradient-recalled echo sequence, where the relative phase shift can be determined by calculating the difference between the maps during heating and preheating.[28,37,38]

Between each sonication, updated anatomic MR imaging is acquired to allow for intraoperative modification of the treatment plan to account for treatment-induced changes in the gland volume. Postablation, dynamic contrast-enhanced (DCE) MR imaging confirms treatment coverage and assesses the devascularized nonviable treatment area (**Figs. 3** and **4**).

MR-GUIDED FOCUSED ULTRASOUND EVIDENCE

During the last 10 years, different phase I and II clinical trials have shown that MRgFUS FT is a safe treatment option with good quality of life outcomes and oncologic response in men with PCa.[7,31,39–42] The main outcomes of these studies are summarized in **Table 2**. The initial proof of principle study reporting preliminary experience of using MRgFUS for FT in localized PCa was that of Napoli and colleagues in 2013.[39] They enrolled 5 patients with unifocal, biopsy-proven PCa evident on MR imaging who underwent ablation with subsequent open radical prostatectomy. The average procedure time was 84 minutes, with a mean maximum temperature of 81.2 C, and a total of 7 to 11 sonications. No severe surgical-related complications were documented. The final histopathology reports showed extensive coagulative necrosis in the ablation zone without residual tumor tissue within or around the treatment area, demonstrating the feasibility of MRgFUS ablation for localized PCa with no significant short-term complications.

Subsequently, Tay and colleagues[42] studied the safety, feasibility, and functional outcomes in 14 patients with low-risk PCa (clinical stage <T2a with Gleason score ≥3 + 3), with a mean age of 62.8 years, a mean prostate volume of 31.5 mL and a mean PSA level of 8.3 ng/dL. All patients underwent MRgFUS focal ablation and follow-up included PSA levels and Expanded Prostate Index Composite questionnaire at 1, 3, 6, 9, 12, 18, and 24 months, as well as mpMR imaging plus transperineal mapping biopsy at 6 and 24 months after treatment. The authors reported good tolerance of the procedure in general, with self-limiting hematuria being the most common early adverse effect. Functional outcomes, particularly related to sexual activity and urinary symptoms, showed insignificant impairment during the first month which normalized at the third month and thereafter. No significant complications were reported, and at 3 months, PSA decreased by a median of 38.8%. However, at 6 months, PSA increased to greater than 10 ng/mL in 6 patients and template biopsy revealed cancer outside the treatment field in 6 men, only 1 with GG2. Twelve of the 14 patients completed the 24 month follow-up; PSA remained low at 2 years in most of the patients, and template biopsy detected PCa in 8 men, 2 with GG2 or greater.

In 2018, Ghai and colleagues[41] included a total of 8 patients (aged 51–68 years), with PSA of 10 ng/mL or less, tumour involving one half of one lobe (cT2a) or less, Gleason score 7 (4 + 3) or less, and prostate volume range of 25 to 50 cc, who underwent MRgFUS. They included a total of 10 lesions (6 GG1 lesions, 2 GG2, and 2 GG3). In this phase I study, the patients were followed for 6 months after the treatment, and their results supported the feasibility and safety of the therapy with good short-term oncologic outcomes. No adverse events occurred during the perioperative period,

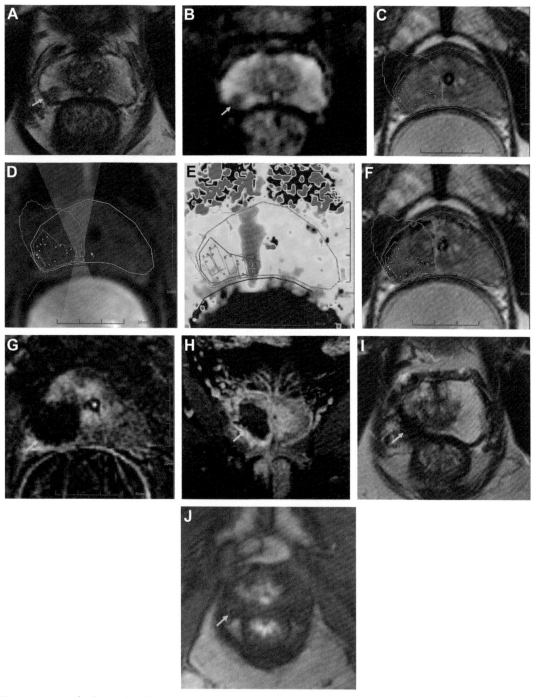

Fig. 3. Imaging findings of a 62 year old patient with biopsy-proven Gleason 7 (3 + 4) prostate cancer. (*A*) Pre-treatment axial T2W fast spin–echo MR imaging (repetition time [TR]/echo time [TE], 3010/125) and (*B*) ADC map image, acquired on a 3T Siemens Skyra Fit scanner, showing the tumor in the right mid gland peripheral zone (*arrows*). (*C*) Intraoperative MR imaging obtained on a 1.5 T GE Excite Twinspeed scanner (GE Healthcare) showing the contoured rectal wall (red *line*), prostate margin (blue outline), and region of interest (orange outline). (*D*) Intraoperative MR imaging showing a focused US beam path (blue) overlaid on the treatment plan. The rectangular boxes within the region of interest illustrate each sonication spot. (*E*) MR imaging thermography image during treatment showing heat deposition color coded in red overlaid on the sonication spot. (*F*) Accumulated thermal dose map image at end of treatment depicting the predicted area of thermal damage color coded in blue. (*G*) Axial precontrast, and (*H*) axial gadovist-enhanced MR imaging obtained immediately

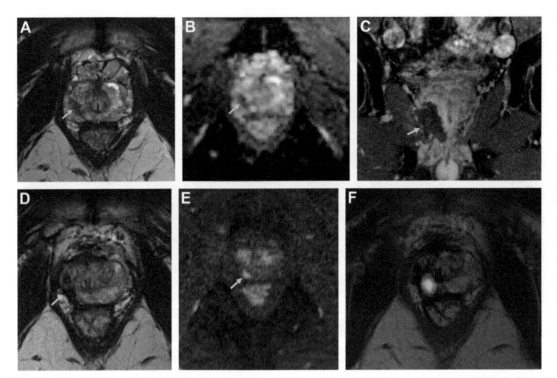

Fig. 4. Imaging findings of a 66 year old patient with biopsy-proven Gleason 7 (3 + 4) prostate cancer. (*A*) Pretreatment axial T2W fast spin–echo MR imaging (TR/TE, 3010/125) and (*B*) ADC map image, acquired on a 3T Siemens Skyra Fit scanner (Siemens Healthcare), showing the tumor in the right mid gland peripheral zone (*arrows*). (*C*) Axial gadovist-enhanced MR imaging obtained immediately posttreatment showing the devascularized ablated volume (*arrows*). (*D*) Corresponding T2W fast spin–echo MR imaging (TR/TE, 3910/97) obtained 6 months posterior to the ablation on the same scanner, showing involution and volume loss at the treated area (*arrow*). (*E*) Corresponding dynamic postcontrast (DCE) image showing early enhancement at the treatment site, suggesting residual disease. (*F*) Correlative (2-(3-{1-carboxy-5-[(6-[18F]fluoro-pyridine-3-carbonyl)-amino]-pentyl}-ureido)-pentanedioic acid [18F-DCFPyL] targeting prostate-specific membrane antigen (PSMA) PET/MR imaging showing focal increased uptake at the site of residual disease. Posterior targeted biopsy of the treatment zone confirmed GG2 tumor.

all patients were discharged within 4 hours of treatment, and none of them required pads for incontinence at any point. Functional outcomes were evaluated according to the International Prostate Symptom Score (IPSS) and the International Index of Erectile Function (IIEF-15) scores. IPSS is designed to evaluate the frequency and severity of lower urinary tract symptoms in men (ie, incomplete emptying, frequency, intermittency, urgency, weak stream, straining, and nocturia), with scores ranging from 0 to 35 to categorize symptoms into mild, moderate, or severe.[43] IIEF-15 assesses erectile function and overall sexual health through a standardized questionnaire with 5 domains (erectile function, orgasmic function, sexual desire,

intercourse satisfaction, and overall satisfaction), with a total score ranging from 5 to 75, offering a comprehensive evaluation of sexual well-being.[44] In 7 patients included in the study, the IPSS showed no significant change between baseline and 6 months, except for 1 patient who experienced a more than 5 point increase in the score due to bilateral peripheral zone ablation. Among the patients with available baseline data for the IIEF-15, scores remained significantly unchanged for 6 out of 7 men between baseline and 6 months posttherapy. However, one patient experienced a notable drop in IIEF-5 score, attributed to urinary tract infection and prostatitis following Foley's catheter removal (Clavien–Dindo grade II). All treated lesions were

---

posttreatment showing the devascularized ablated volume (*arrows*). (*I*) Corresponding T2W fast spin-echo MR imaging (TR/TE, 3910/97) obtained 24 months posterior to the ablation on the same scanner, showing involution and volume loss at the treated area (*arrow*). (*J*) Corresponding dynamic postcontrast (DCE) image does not show any focus of early or contemporaneous enhancement at the treatment site or margins. Findings from a targeted biopsy of the treatment zone and the rest of the gland were negative.

Table 2
MR-guided focused ultrasound studies for prostate cancer

Study Characteristics	Napoli et al.[39] 2013	Tay et al.[42] 2017	Ghai, et al.[41] 2018	Ehdaie et al.[7] 2022	Ghai et al.[45] 2024
Number of patients (n)	n=5	n=14	n=8 patients (10 lesions)	n=101	n=44
Study objective	Proof of principle study (single center)	Phase I safety and efficacy study (single center)	Phase I safety and efficacy study (single center)	Phase II safety, functional and oncological outcomes (multicenter)	Phase II safety, functional and oncological outcomes (single center)
Inclusion criteria	• Men who had consented to radical prostatectomy for PCa, Unifocal, biopsy-proven PCa on mpMR imaging (GG1 [n=3]) GG2 (n=2)	• Age 50–75 y • GG1 • ≤cT2a • Index tumor ≤10 cc • Maximum of 2 positive zones on biopsy or MR-identifiable tumors or a combination of the two	• PSA ≤10 ng/mL • ≤cT2a • ≤GG3 (GG1 [n=6]) GG 2 (n=2) GG 3 (n=2)	• Age >50 y • Unilateral, organ-confined, visible on mpMR imaging • Intermediate-risk cancer (GG2 or GG3, stage ≤T2) • PSA ≤20 ng/mL	• Age ≥50 y • Unifocal, organ-confined, <20 mm max length, • Intermediate-risk PCa (GG2 or GG3) PSA ≤20 ng/mL • Life expectancy >10 y
Study duration	Radical prostatectomy in 7–14 d (mean 9 d)	2 y	6 mo	2 y	2 y
Complications	No technical difficulties related to MRgFUS ablation during surgery	Seven men had Clavien-Dindo grade 1–2 complications (1 acute urinary retention, 1 epididymo-orchitis 5 self-limiting hematuria)	Not reported	• 1 patient with urinary tract infection	• 1 patient with persistent pelvic pain
PSA	N/A	• Median decrease by 2.9 ng/mL at 6 mo	• Mean decrease by 1.66 ng/mL at 6 mo	• Mean decrease by 2.6 ng/mL at 24 mo	• Median decrease by 3.7 ng/mL at 24 mo

(continued on next page)

Table 2
(continued)

Study Characteristics	Napoli et al.[39] 2013	Tay et al.[42] 2017	Ghai, et al.[41] 2018	Ehdaie et al.[7] 2022	Ghai et al.[45] 2024
Functional outcomes	N/A	• No significant change in urinary symptom and sexual function scores at 2 y	• Quality of life parameters stable between baseline and 6 mo in 6 out of 8 patients	• IIEF-15 score slightly worse (−3.5) at 24 mo: • No significant change in IPSS scores	• No significant decline in IIEF-15 and IPSS scores
Oncologic outcomes	Extensive coagulative necrosis at ablation site. No residual viable tumor in the ablation area or margins	At 6 mo: • 6 patients with ≥GG1 (1 with ≥GG2) At 24 mo: • 8 out of 12 patients in field/adjacent recurrence (3 with ≥GG2)	At 6 mo: • 3 out of 10 sites GG1 disease • 1 out of 10 site GG4 disease	At 24 mo: • 78 out of 89 (88%) free of csPCa (≥GG2) at the treated site; and 59 out of 98 (60%) in the entire gland	At 24 mo: • 39 out of 43 (91%) free of csPCa (≥GG2) at the treated area; and 36 out of 43 (84%) in entire gland

Abbreviations: csPCa, clinically significant prostate cancer; GG, Gleason Grade Group; IIEF-15, International Index of Erectile Function-15; IPSS, International Prostate Symptom Score; mpMR imaging, multiparametric MR imaging; PSA, prostate-specific antigen.

negative on mpMR imaging, and 60% of the targeted lesions were negative on MR imaging - guided biopsy with one man with persistent csPCa (≥GG2).

More recently, Ehdaie and colleagues,[7] conducted a single-arm, multicenter, phase II study among 8 health care centers in the United States, with excellent 6 month and 24 month oncological outcomes at the treatment site. They included 101 patients with previously untreated unilateral intermediate-risk PCa (79 with GG2 disease and 22 with GG3 PCa), with a median age of 63 years and median PSA of 5.7 ng/mL, who underwent MRgFUS. At 6 month assessment, PSA mean decrease was −3.0 ng/mL (95% CI −3.6 to −2.4), and 96 out of 101 patients (95% CI 89–98) exhibited no evidence of GG2 or higher PCa in the treated area on MR imaging-targeted and systematic biopsy. At 24 months, PSA measurements showed a slight increase when compared to 6 months, and MR imaging-guided biopsy revealed no evidence of GG2 or higher grade lesions in 78 out of 89 patients (88%). IIEF-15 scores were slightly worse with a mean score difference of −3.5 (95% CI −5.4 to −1.6), and the probability of functional erections decreased, for example, with 4 out of 40 men who had functional erections at baseline, reporting severe erectile dysfunction.

A further phase II trial by Ghai and colleagues,[31,45] evaluated the 2 year oncological and functional outcomes in a group of 44 patients with unifocal csPCa. They included men aged 50 years or older with unifocal, localized, intermediate-risk PCa (36 patients with GG2 at baseline, and 8 patients with GG3), PSA of 20 ng/mL or less. There were no major complications. Functional assessment was obtained with IPSS and IIEF-15 questionnaires and PSA measurements were assessed at 6 weeks and 5, 12, 18, and 24 months. MpMR imaging followed by targeted fusion biopsy was performed at 5 and 24 months following treatment. The median PSA level at 2 years decreased in most patients. The 5 month biopsy showed residual csPCa (≥GG2) at the treatment site in 7% of the patients. Similarly, of the 42 patients who underwent 2 year biopsy, 7% showed csPCa at the treatment site; overall, 9% of men exhibited in-field, persistent csPCa over 2 years, while 91% remained free of csPCa at the treatment site. At the 24 month follow-up, 42 men completed the IPSS and IIEF-15 questionnaires. The median IPSS score showed no significant change and no participants reported pad use at 24 months. For erectile function, no significant difference was observed in overall IIEF-15 scores between baseline and 24 months.

MR-GUIDED FOCUSED ULTRASOUND, IMAGING FINDINGS, AND FOLLOW-UP

Imaging follow-up after FT should be performed with mpMR imaging, in accordance with the available expert consensus.[4] Additionally, the expert panel also recommends that mpMR imaging followed by biopsy should be performed within the first year of treatment in all patients. Immediate posttreatment scans show gland edema, architectural distortion, and hemorrhage secondary to coagulative necrosis in the treated area and adjacent tissues. The ablation zone will manifest on DCE images as a nonperfused volume, which can persist for up to 1 month. After 3 to 6 months, MR imaging may show atrophic and retractile changes at the level of the ablation site, representing scarring and fibrosis.[36,38] Findings suggestive of treatment failure and/or recurrent disease include early contrast enhancement in the treated lesion or its margins, and the combination of hyperintense signal on high B value DW image and hypointense signal on the apparent diffusion coefficient (ADC) map[46] (see **Figs. 3** and **4**).

Giganti and colleagues[47] have proposed an initial scoring system for follow-up with mpMR imaging, based on a single institutional experience called "prostate imaging after focal ablation." However, this system lacks validation, is not routinely used in current practice, and there are ongoing efforts to determine a system in accordance with the prostate imaging reporting and data system (PI-RADS) and prostate imaging recurrence reporting (PI-RR) international consensus-based guidelines.[48] Nontreated areas of the prostate should be assessed as per PI-RADS v2.1 recommendations for detection of de novo disease.

SUMMARY

In conclusion, studies examining MRgFUS as a therapeutic modality for intermediate-risk localized PCa have demonstrated promising results in terms of both oncological efficacy and functional outcomes. The noninvasive nature of MRgFUS, coupled with its ability to precisely target and ablate prostate tumors, highlights its potential as a valuable alternative or complementary approach to existing treatments. The favorable outcomes observed in these studies underscore the importance and validates the efficacy and safety of MRgFUS in PCa management. As we move forward, MRgFUS stands as a pioneer innovation in FT for PCa, offering a potential paradigm shift toward personalized and minimally invasive intervention with the potential to enhance patient outcomes and quality of life.

CLINICS CARE POINTS

- There are no universal eligibility criteria for FT to date. In our experience, ideal candidates are those with MR imaging-visible lesions measuring up to 15 mm, clinical stage T1c to T2a, GG2 or GG3 disease, PSA level less than 15 to 20 ng/mL, and life expectancy greater than 5 to 10 years.

- MR imaging-guided FT advantages includ targeted approach, enabling a smaller and precise ablation volume; smaller ablation volumes have shown better functional outcomes.

- MRgFUS FT is a safe treatment option with good quality of life outcomes in men with localized PCa. Multiple studies have shown that MRgFUS FT is associated with minimal short-term complications and acceptable functional outcomes, including urinary and sexual function.

- MRgFUS FT has shown promising oncologic outcomes in terms of tumor control. Studies have reported a decrease in PSA levels post-treatment, indicating effective tumor ablation. Additionally, imaging-guided biopsies have shown negative or reduced cancer detection rates in the treated area over the short to medium term. However, a subset of patients may exhibit residual or recurrent cancer, highlighting the importance of long-term follow-up and ongoing monitoring.

REFERENCES

1. Alabousi M, Ghai S, Haider MA. MRI-guided Minimally Invasive Focal Therapies for Prostate Cancer. Radiology 2023;309(3). https://doi.org/10.1148/radiol.230431.

2. Wang L, Lu B, He M, et al. Prostate Cancer Incidence and Mortality: Global Status and Temporal Trends in 89 Countries From 2000 to 2019. Front Public Health 2022;10. https://doi.org/10.3389/fpubh.2022.811044.

3. Heard JR, Naser-Tavakolian A, Nazmifar M, et al. Focal prostate cancer therapy in the era of multiparametric MRI: a review of options and outcomes. Prostate Cancer Prostatic Dis 2023;26(2):218–27.

4. Lebastchi AH, George AK, Polascik TJ, et al. Standardized Nomenclature and Surveillance Methodologies After Focal Therapy and Partial Gland Ablation for Localized Prostate Cancer: An International Multidisciplinary Consensus. Eur Urol 2020;78(3):371–8.

5. Tay KJ, Scheltema MJ, Ahmed HU, et al. Patient selection for prostate focal therapy in the era of active surveillance: an International Delphi Consensus Project. Prostate Cancer Prostatic Dis 2017;20(3):294–9.

6. Eastham JA, Boorjian SA, Kirkby E. Clinically Localized Prostate Cancer: AUA/ASTRO Guideline. J Urol 2022;208(3):505–7.

7. Ehdaie B, Tempany CM, Holland F, et al. MRI-guided focused ultrasound focal therapy for patients with intermediate-risk prostate cancer: a phase 2b, multicentre study. Lancet Oncol 2022;23(7):910–8.

8. Morash C, Tey R, Agbassi C, et al. Active surveillance for the management of localized prostate cancer: Guideline recommendations. Canadian Urological Association Journal 2015;9(5–6):171.

9. MRI-guided Minimally Invasive Focal Therapies for Prostate Cancer. Available at: https://pubs.rsna.org/doi/epdf/10.1148/radiol.230431. [Accessed 9 December 2023].

10. Ghai S, Perlis N. Beyond the AJR: MRI-Guided Focused Ultrasound Focal Therapy for Intermediate-Risk Prostate Cancer. Am J Roentgenol 2023;220(4):910.

11. Mouraviev V, Mayes JM, Polascik TJ. Pathologic basis of focal therapy for early-stage prostate cancer. Nat Rev Urol 2009;6(4):205–15.

12. Ong S, Chen K, Grummet J, et al. Guidelines of guidelines: focal therapy for prostate cancer, is it time for consensus? BJU Int 2023;131(1):20–31.

13. van Luijtelaar A, Greenwood BM, Ahmed HU, et al. Focal laser ablation as clinical treatment of prostate cancer: report from a Delphi consensus project. World J Urol 2019;37(10):2147–53.

14. Mjaess G, Peltier A, Roche JB, et al. A Novel Nomogram to Identify Candidates for Focal Therapy Among Patients with Localized Prostate Cancer Diagnosed via Magnetic Resonance Imaging–Targeted and Systematic Biopsies: A European Multicenter Study. Eur Urol Focus 2023;9(6):992–9.

15. Javier-DesLoges J, Dall'Era MA, Brisbane W, et al. The state of focal therapy in the treatment of prostate cancer: the university of California collaborative (UC-Squared) consensus statement. Prostate Cancer Prostatic Dis 2023. https://doi.org/10.1038/s41391-023-00702-1.

16. Huber PM, Afzal N, Arya M, et al. Focal HIFU therapy for anterior compared to posterior prostate cancer lesions. World J Urol 2021;39(4):1115–9.

17. Perera M, Krishnananthan N, Lindner U, et al. An update on focal therapy for prostate cancer. Nat Rev Urol 2016;13(11):641–53.

18. Bakavicius A, Marra G, Macek P, et al. Available evidence on HIFU for focal treatment of prostate cancer: a systematic review ARTICLE INFO IBJU | SYSTEMATIC REVIEW OF FOCAL HIFU IN PROSTATE CANCER. Int Braz J Urol 2022;48(2):263–74.

19. Chin YF, Lynn N. Systematic Review of Focal and Salvage Cryotherapy for Prostate Cancer. Cureus 2022. https://doi.org/10.7759/cureus.26400.

20. Xue Q, Zhang J, Jiao J, et al. Photodynamic therapy for prostate cancer: Recent advances, challenges and opportunities. Front Oncol 2022. https://doi.org/10.3389/fonc.2022.980239.

21. Walser E, Nance A, Ynalvez L, et al. Focal Laser Ablation of Prostate Cancer: Results in 120 Patients with Low- to Intermediate-Risk Disease. J Vasc Intervent Radiol 2019;30(3):401–9.e2.

22. Paxton M, Barbalat E, Perlis N, et al. Role of multiparametric MRI in long-term surveillance following focal laser ablation of prostate cancer. Br J Radiol 2022; 95(1131). https://doi.org/10.1259/bjr.20210414.

23. Blazevski A, Scheltema MJ, Yuen B, et al. Oncological and Quality-of-life Outcomes Following Focal Irreversible Electroporation as Primary Treatment for Localised Prostate Cancer: A Biopsy-monitored Prospective Cohort. Eur Urol Oncol 2020;3(3): 283–90.

24. Jolesz FA. MRI-guided focused ultrasound surgery. Annu Rev Med 2009;60:417–30.

25. Wu F, Wang ZB, Chen WZ, et al. Extracorporeal high intensity focused ultrasound ablation in the treatment of 1038 patients with solid carcinomas in China: an overview. Ultrason Sonochem 2004;11(3–4): 149–54.

26. Stabile A, Giganti F, Rosenkrantz AB, et al. Multiparametric MRI for prostate cancer diagnosis: current status and future directions. Nat Rev Urol 2019;17(1):41–61.

27. Alabousi M, Ghai S. Magnetic resonance imaging-guided ultrasound ablation for prostate cancer – A contemporary review of performance. Front Oncol 2023;12:1069518.

28. Adamo DA, Greenwood BM, Ghanouni P, et al. MR Imaging-Guided Prostate Cancer Therapies. Radiol Clin North Am 2024;62(1):121–33.

29. Masoom SN, Sundaram KM, Ghanouni P, et al. Real-Time MRI-Guided Prostate Interventions. Cancers 2022;14(8):1860.

30. Faure Walker NA, Norris JM, Shah TT, et al. A comparison of time taken to return to baseline erectile function following focal and whole gland ablative therapies for localized prostate cancer: A systematic review. Urol Oncol: Seminars and Original Investigations 2018;36(2):67–76.

31. Ghai S, Finelli A, Corr K, et al. MRI-guided Focused ultrasound ablation for localized intermediate-risk prostate cancer: Early results of a phase II trial. Radiology 2021;298(3):695–703.

32. Pooli A, Johnson DC, Shirk J, et al. Predicting Pathological Tumor Size in Prostate Cancer Based on Multiparametric Prostate Magnetic Resonance Imaging and Preoperative Findings. J Urol 2021; 205(2):444–51.

33. Le Nobin J, Rosenkrantz AB, Villers A, et al. Image Guided Focal Therapy for Magnetic Resonance Imaging Visible Prostate Cancer: Defining a 3-Dimensional Treatment Margin Based on Magnetic Resonance Imaging Histology Co-Registration Analysis. J Urol 2015;194(2):364–70.

34. Priester A, Natarajan S, Khoshnoodi P, et al. Magnetic Resonance Imaging Underestimation of Prostate Cancer Geometry: Use of Patient Specific Molds to Correlate Images with Whole Mount Pathology. J Urol 2017;197(2):320–6.

35. Ghai S, Louis AS, Vliet M Van, et al. Real-time MRI-guided focused ultrasound for focal therapy of locally confined low-risk prostate cancer: Feasibility and preliminary outcomes. Am J Roentgenol 2015; 205(2):W177–84.

36. Patel P, Mathew MS, Trilisky I, et al. Multiparametric MR imaging of the prostate after treatment of prostate cancer. Radiographics 2018;38(2):437–49.

37. Chen WH, Sanghvi NT, Carlson R, et al. Validation of tissue change monitoring (TCM) on the Sonablate® 500 during high intensity focused ultrasound (HIFU) treatment of prostate cancer with real-time thermometry. AIP Conf Proc 2012;1481(1):53–8.

38. Tayebi S, Verma S, Sidana A. Real-Time and Delayed Imaging of Tissue and Effects of Prostate Tissue Ablation. Curr Urol Rep 2023;24(10):477–89.

39. Napoli A, Anzidei M, De Nunzio C, et al. Real-time magnetic resonance-guided high-intensity focused ultrasound focal therapy for localised prostate cancer: Preliminary experience. Eur Urol 2013;63(2): 395–8.

40. von Hardenberg J, Borkowetz A, Siegel F, et al. Potential Candidates for Focal Therapy in Prostate Cancer in the Era of Magnetic Resonance Imaging–targeted Biopsy: A Large Multicenter Cohort Study. Eur Urol Focus 2021;7(5):1002–10.

41. Ghai S, Perlis N, Lindner U, et al. Magnetic resonance guided focused high frequency ultrasound ablation for focal therapy in prostate cancer – phase 1 trial. Eur Radiol 2018;28(10):4281–7.

42. Tay KJ, Cheng CWS, Lau WKO, et al. Focal therapy for prostate cancer with in-bore MR-guided focused ultrasound: Two-year follow-up of a phase i trial - Complications and functional outcomes. Radiology 2017;285(2):620–8.

43. Gewanter RM, Sandhu JS, Tin MAAL, et al. Assessment of Patients With Prostate Cancer and Their Understanding of the International Prostate Symptom Score Questionnaire. Adv Radiat Oncol 2023;8: 101200.

44. Neijenhuijs KI, Holtmaat K, Aaronson NK, et al. The International Index of Erectile Function (IIEF)—A Systematic Review of Measurement Properties. J Sex Med 2019;16(7):1078–91.

45. Ghai S, Antonio A, Corr K, et al. MRI-guided focused ultrasound focal therapy for intermediate-

risk prostate cancer: final results from a 2-Year phase II clinical trial. Radiology 2024;310(3): e231473.

46. Paxton M, Barbalat E, Perlis N, et al. INNOVATIONS IN PROSTATE CANCER SPECIAL FEATURE : FULL PAPER Role of multiparametric MRI in long-term sur- veillance following focal laser ablation of prostate cancer 1. Br J Radiol 2022. https://doi.org/10.1259/bjr.20210414.

47. Giganti F, Allen C, Emberton M, et al. Prostate Imag- ing Quality (PI-QUAL): A New Quality Control Scoring System for Multiparametric Magnetic Reso- nance Imaging of the Prostate from the PRECISION trial. Eur Urol Oncol 2020;3(5):615–9.

48. Abreu-Gomez J, Haider M, Re Ghai S, et al. Prostate Imaging After Focal Ablation (PI-FAB): A Proposal

for a Scoring System for Multiparametric MRI of the Prostate After Focal Therapy. Eur Urol Oncol. In press. https://doi.org/10.1016/j.euo.2023.04.007. Eur Urol Oncol 2023. https://doi.org/10.1016/J.EUO.2023.07.015.

49. Epstein JI, Egevad L, Amin MB, et al. The 2014 inter- national society of urological pathology (ISUP) consensus conference on gleason grading of pros- tatic carcinoma definition of grading patterns and proposal for a new grading system. Am J Surg Pathol 2016;40(2):244–52.

50. Van Leenders GJLH, Van Der Kwast TH, Grignon DJ, et al. The 2019 International Society of Urological Pathology (ISUP) Consensus Conference on Grading of Prostatic Carcinoma. Am J Surg Pathol 2020;44(8):E87–99.

MR-guided Focused Ultrasound for Musculoskeletal Applications

Christin A. Tiegs-Heiden, MD

KEYWORDS

- MR-guided focused ultrasound • Musculoskeletal • Bone metastasis • Osteoid osteoma
- Osteoarthritis

KEY POINTS

- MR-guided focused ultrasound (MRgFUS) can be used for the ablation of both benign and malignant bone and soft tissue lesions.
- MRgFUS is US Food and Drug Administration approved and has the CE mark for the treatment of osteoid osteoma and painful bone metastases; it also has the CE mark for the treatment of lumbar facet joints.
- MRgFUS is also being evaluated for sacroiliac joint pain, knee osteoarthritis, desmoid fibromatosis, peripheral nerve ablation, and vascular malformations.

INTRODUCTION

MR-guided focused ultrasound (MRgFUS) combines accurate targeting and real-time thermal monitoring to provide precise tissue ablation.[1] These benefits make it a promising therapeutic option for a wide variety of musculoskeletal applications, including bone and soft tissue lesions, both benign and malignant.

Focused ultrasound has the CE mark for the treatment of osteoid osteoma, painful bone metastases, and facet joint osteoarthritis.[2] It has US Food and Drug Administration approval for painful bone metastases and osteoid osteoma.[2]

The purpose of this review is to describe the current state of MRgFUS for musculoskeletal applications and highlighting key evidence and areas for future research.

PAINFUL BONE METASTASES

Osseous metastatic disease may result in significant morbidity to affected patients, including pain, decreased mobility, and pathologic fracture.[3] Radiation therapy is the current standard of care for the palliative treatment of painful bone metastases but has a 20% to 40% failure rate for pain reduction, an up to 4 week latency period, known side effects, and potential for pain relapse.[4–7] Thus, thermal radiation methods including MRgFUS have been evaluated as an alternate treatment option.[6] Such options may be particularly important for radiation-resistant cancers such as melanoma, colorectal, and renal cell carcinoma.[4]

MRgFUS has been shown to be safe and effective in the palliative treatment of painful bone metastases.[4] Two systematic review and meta-analyses exist that evaluate its efficacy and safety, one including 33 studies with 1082 patients[4] and the other 15 studies and 362 patients.[6] These analyses found a pooled response rate of 77% to 79%.[4,6] One reported a −3.8 and −4.4 difference in a numerical rating scale (NRS) pain score at 1 and 3 months, respectively.[4] The other found a mean reduction in pain score of 4.22 at 5 to 14 weeks.[6] Opioid use decreased after treatment, evidenced by reduction in oral morphine equivalent daily dose scores and 55.8%/33.0% rates of stopping/reducing pain medications.[4,6] Only 5 studies evaluated the quality-of-life following MRgFUS, but all showed improvement.[4] The impact on functional ability is not well understood,

Division of Musculoskeletal Radiology, Mayo Clinic, 200 1st Street Southwest, Rochester, MN 55905, USA
E-mail address: tiegsheiden.christin@mayo.edu

Magn Reson Imaging Clin N Am 32 (2024) 641–650
https://doi.org/10.1016/j.mric.2024.02.006

with the few available studies showing mixed results.[4]

In patients who had previously undergone external beam radiation, 74% achieved pain relief with MRgFUS, compared to 58% response rate in a meta-analysis of re-irradiation therapy.[4,8] Unlike radiation, there are no additive risks of repeat MRgFUS treatments.[4]

Pooled rate of high- and low-grade adverse events following MRgFUS was 0.9% and 5.9%, respectively, from 26 total studies in the larger meta-analysis.[4] The other meta-analysis reported higher rates, with major complications in 1.42% and minor complications in 26.4%.[6] Major complications/high-grade events included fractures, third-degree skin burn, hip flexor neuropathy, and sciatic nerve injury.[6] Rate of postradiation fracture has been reported at 1%.[9]

MRgFUS had 3% incidence of acute pain flare.[4] This is considerably lower than with stereotactic and external beam radiation, where incidence is reported to be 30% to 43%.[9,10]

Pain relief achieved by MRgFUS is believed to be largely a result of denervation of the treated periosteum.[7,11] Additionally, MRgFUS may result in tumor debulking, a decrease in the release of chemical mediators and osteoclast-mediated osteolysis, and induce skeletal remodeling.[7] MRgFUS is thought to stimulate bone healing, with some studies reporting new bone formation at the treatment site.[11,12] It has also been shown that levels of circulating tumor-secreted immunosuppressive cytokines are lower after MRgFUS, which could potentially improve antitumor immunity.[13]

Of note, one study reported difficulty in achieving ablative temperatures greater than 55°C and pain relief in tumors with complete cortical destruction and therefore hypothesized that higher energy sonications may be necessary for such lesions.[14]

OSTEOID OSTEOMA AND OSTEOBLASTOMA

Osteoid osteoma is a benign painful bone tumor with characteristic imaging features, most commonly affecting individuals under the age of 30 years.[15] Conservative management is typically not a viable option in these patients due to inadequate pain relief and side effects of medication.[16] Currently, computed tomography (CT)-guided percutaneous radiofrequency (RF) or laser ablation is considered the standard intervention for these lesions.[16,17] These minimally invasive procedures carry minor risks, including damage to surrounding tissues, bleeding, and infection, and require exposure to radiation.[17]

MRgFUS has gained attention as a noninvasive and radiation-free treatment option for osteoid osteoma.[16] A recent systematic review and meta-analysis of MRgFUS for osteoid osteoma included 15 studies with 353 total patients published between 2012 and 2022, mostly single-arm trials.[17] Lesions were located in a variety of non-spinal locations, the majority in the femur (n = 100).[17] Pooled success rate was 92.8%, with a successful treatment defined as complete pain relief, and 5.4% of patients underwent secondary interventions.[17] Only 3 complications were reported, all from the same study, and all being minor thermal injuries at the ablation site.[17,18]

To be amenable to MRgFUS, an osteoid osteoma must be visible on noncontrast MR imaging, greater than 1 cm from the skin, growth plate, and neurovascular bundles, and accessible to the FUS beam.[16] Lesions in the skull and non-sacral spine are not yet being treated with MRgFUS.[16] Thick cortical bone overlying the nidus may reduce the efficacy of MRgFUS, as it is challenging for the ultrasound beam to penetrate to deeper lesions.[19,20]

Bone requires less energy to produce heating than soft tissue lesions.[16] In one prospective study of 29 treatments, a mean of 7 ± 3 sonications and mean acoustic energy of 1180 ± 736 Joules (J) were used.[21] This is higher than in the initial description, which utilized a mean of 866 J.[22] One group recommended placing a cluster of sonications around the nidus to maximize energy deposition within it.[16] They also recommended slowly increasing energy starting at 40 to 60 W for 20 to 30 s until the target bone surface temperature measures or exceeds 65°C.[16]

Several studies have compared MRgFUS to CT-guided RF ablation, consisting of 9, 13, and 48 matched patients.[18,20,23] All showed comparable pain response and functional recovery between the 2 treatment modalities.[18,20,23] Total intraprocedural and recovery time was not significantly different between the groups in one study.[23] A phase III trial comparing MRgFUS and RF ablation (RFA) is currently ongoing (ClinicalTrials.gov ID: NCT02923011).

MRgFUS of the larger but otherwise histologically identical osteoblastoma has also been reported.[19] In a retrospective study of 6 patients, intra-articular osteoblastoma was successfully treated with MRgFUS in all cases, with reduction in pain and improvement in function.[24] One consideration is that MRgFUS lacks the ability to biopsy at the time of procedure, so should be limited to clearly radiographically benign lesions given the rare occurrence of malignant transformation of osteoblastoma.[25]

Motivated by the very low risk of pathologic fracture after RFA, one study examined bone density changes following MRgFUS treatment of osteoid osteoma and osteoblastoma on follow-up CT.[26] Given the lack of mechanical penetration, MRgFUS could potentially reduce this risk.[16] Thirty-six patients (31 osteoid osteoma and 5 intra-articular osteoblastomas) were followed for a mean of 18 months.[26] Bone density within the lesion itself increased after treatment with resolution of previously seen osteolysis, while normal surrounding bone did not change significantly.[26] This study only evaluated bone density changes in the long-term following the procedure, not acutely.

OTHER BENIGN LESIONS

In one article describing the experience of a single institution, the authors reported that they have treated 12 "benign epiphyseal lesions" (described as 2 periosteal chondromas, 1 fibroangioma, 6 fibroosseous lesions, 2 fibromixoangiomas, and 1 osteoblastoma).[27] They report response in all patients, with 90% improvement in visual analog scale and no lesion progression, resolution of any surrounding edema and enhancement at 12 month follow-up.[27] The same institution reported safe and effective treatment in 14 intra-articular benign bone lesions.[28] No other literature was found regarding the aforementioned entities.

FACET JOINTS

In patients with low back pain, the prevalence of lumbar facet joint pain is typically reported to be 10% to 20% in high-quality studies.[29,30] Fluoroscopically guided RFA of the medial branch nerves is the treatment of choice for patients who have failed a 3 month trial of conservative measures.[29,30] A 2015 Cochrane analysis and separate 2015 review both found moderate evidence for the effectiveness of RFA for short-term relief of low back pain, and low evidence for longer term relief.[29,31]

Phantom and animal experiments have shown that MRgFUS can successfully ablate the lumbar facet joints without heating the surrounding neural foramen, spinal canal, or vertebral body.[32] Swine models have successfully targeted the proximal medial branch with high-intensity focused ultrasound (HIFU), using MR imaging guidance in one study[33] and fluoroscopic guidance in the other.[33] Transient skin erythema was observed in 2 pigs in one of the studies.[33]

There are relatively few published studies of MRgFUS in patients with lumbar facet joint pain. Several retrospective series have assessed the safety and efficacy of lumbar facet joint MRgFUS in 26,[34] 18 (follow-up data available in 13),[35] and 11 patients.[36] The posterior facet joints were targeted, typically L3-4, L4-5, and L5-S1 bilaterally, with 3 to 4 sonications per joint.[34,35] Energies ranged from 1055 to 1648 J in one study[34] and 450 to 750 J in another.[35] The largest series achieved greater than 3 month pain relief in 60% of patients.[34] Duration of relief ranged from 6 to 34 months, with a mean of 13.3.[34] Higher success rates were seen in the subgroup of patients who had at least some relief to prior RFA.[34] In another study, patients reported 60.2%/51.2% mean decrease in average/worst NRS score at 6 months and improved functional disability.[35] The final study reported response rate of 64% at 1 week and 1 month and 82% at 3 months.[36] Median NRS score significantly decreased, from 8 (4 to 9) to 3 (0 to 7) at the final follow-up at 3 months.[36] There were no significant treatment-related complications reported.[34,35] These studies theorized that the procedure results in denervation of the terminal nerve branches around the facet joint.[34,35] MRgFUS of the lumbar facet joints using this technique is illustrated in **Fig. 1**.

A 10 patient pilot study targeted the medial branch nerve with fluoroscopically guided FUS in patients with chronic facet-mediated low back pain.[37] Success rate was similar to conventional RFA.[37] Similar studies utilizing MR guidance in human subjects are not available.

SACROILIAC JOINTS

The estimated prevalence of sacroiliac (SI) joint pain in patients with low back pain is 25%.[38] Interventional treatment options include steroid injection, RF lateral branch nerve ablation, and joint fusion surgery.[38] In some individuals, variable innervation of the joint can impact the success of traditional RFA.[39] MRgFUS could provide an alternative noninvasive ablation method for SI joint pain.

In a preliminary swine model, 3 animals underwent MRgFUS of the bilateral SI joints.[40] All procedures successfully produced contiguous lesions along both joints; however, in the first case, excessive heating of near-field muscle caused tissue necrosis.[40] Further studies are needed to confirm the feasibility and safety of the procedure, as well as to determine an optimal treatment approach.

KNEE JOINT OSTEOARTHRITIS

Chronic knee pain from osteoarthritis is common in the elderly and may lead to functional disability

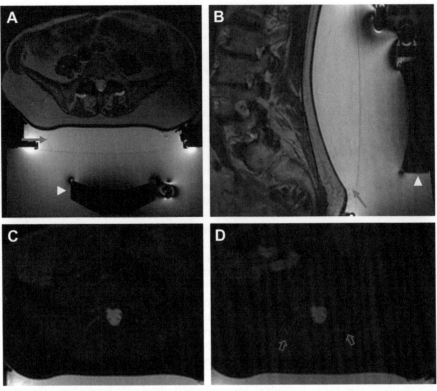

Fig. 1. MRgFUS of painful lumbar facet joints. (*A*, *B*) Planning axial and sagittal T2-weigthed images show the patient lying supine over the transducer (*arrowheads*), with an interposed water bag (*arrows*). The posterior facet joint capsule (blue crescents, A) is the ablation target in this case. T2 fat-saturated images obtained pre- (*C*) and post- (*D*) treatment show the development of a small amount of soft tissue edema along the posterior aspect of the targeted facet joints (*open arrows*).

and reduced quality of life.[1] While total knee arthroplasty is a well-validated treatment option, there are some patients who are unable or unwilling to undergo the procedure.[1] An effective noninvasive option for knee pain could be beneficial for such patients. Based on characteristic tenderness to palpation of the knee joint, it has been hypothesized that MRgFUS ablation of nociceptors and primary afferent sensory nerves about the joint could provide pain relief.[36,41]

There are limited published data on the use of MRgFUS for treatment of knee pain from osteoarthritis. In a case series of 8 patients over 60 years of age with knee osteoarthritis and severe medial knee pain, the authors evaluated the safety and efficacy of MRgFUS using a conformable system.[41] The ablation target was the tibial cortical surface just below the rim osteophyte, near the insertion of the deep medial collateral ligament fibers.[41] Patients were treated with a mean of 12.4 sonications and mean therapeutic energy level of 735 J.[41] Following treatment, visual analog scale (VAS) with waking was reduced by 60% or greater in 6 of 8 patients at 1 month; 4 patients had sustained

relief of at least 6 months.[41] Patients who benefitted also had significantly increased pain pressure threshold (PPT) in the medial knee following treatment, leading the authors to hypothesize that FUS treatment at sites of severe tenderness may relieve knee pain.[41] No adverse events were reported.[41] Follow-up radiographs in treated patients demonstrated subcortical sclerosis underlying the area of treatment.[41]

In a follow-up study, 19 patients aged over 60 years with refractory medial knee pain and Kellgren-Lawrence grade III or IV osteoarthritis were treated with MRgFUS in the area of greatest tenderness.[1] The location of lowest PPT was determined with the use of a handheld algometer; this site was correlated under MRI guidance using an MRI-compatible skin marker and was designated the target for ablation.[1] A 1 cm diameter sonication was placed on the bone surface in this location, avoiding the joint space and popliteal neurovascular bundle with the beam.[1] The treatment utilized local anesthetic and no sedation; however, it is notable that 8 patients used the stop sonication button due to pain, 5 patients used once, and 3 patients used 4 to 6 times, though all patients completed the procedure.[1] Response rate was 68.4% (13 patients) at 3 and 6 months and 73.7% (14 patients) at 1 and 12 months.[1] Mean worst NRS pain score showed continued decline over 12 months and remained significantly reduced at the final follow-up.[1] Western Ontario and McMaster Universities Osteoarthritis Index (WOMAC) scores also remained significantly improved over the follow-up course.[1] Two subjects (10.5%) underwent TKA within 3 months due to lack of sufficient pain relief.[1] There were no major complications, including skin burn.[1] Nearly half of patients showed sclerosis at the treatment site on follow-up CT; however, none developed fracture or collapse, or osteoarthritis progression.[1]

No literature regarding MRgFUS treatment of other painful peripheral joints was identified.

EXTRA-ABDOMINAL DESMOID FIBROMATOSIS

Desmoid fibromatosis is a rare monoclonal mesenchymal tumor, most commonly diagnosed in the second to fourth decades.[42] Given the lack of metastatic potential, management seeks to obtain local tumor control with the lowest possible morbidity and is typically reserved for growing or symptomatic tumors.[42,43] Conventional treatment options include operative resection, radiation therapy, and/or systemic chemotherapy.[43] Recurrence rate following surgery has been reported at 30% to 60%, and morbidity rates from these treatments are also relatively high.[42] As a result, less invasive options such as percutaneous ablation and FUS treatment have gained attention.[42,44] Although recurrence rates remain high, morbidity is lower and these procedures offer the ability for retreatment.[42]

Smaller preliminary studies demonstrated the feasibility of MRgFUS for patients with extra-abdominal desmoid fibromatosis who were not good candidates for excision, radiation, or chemotherapy due to risk of morbidity, prior failure, or refusal.[45] Subsequently, a multicenter retrospective study of 105 patients with 111 tumors was published, including 36 patients who underwent multiple treatments (median 2, range 2 to 5).[46] The majority of these patients had undergone prior treatment.[46] Median tumor volume decreased from 114 mL initially (median 85 mL targeted by treatment), to a total/viable volume of 51 mL (34% decrease) and 29 mL (64% decrease), respectively, at last follow-up (median 15 months, range 11 to 20 months).[46] Greatest decrease in total tumor volume was seen at 16 months, and of viable tumor volume at 11 months.[46] When

residual viable tumor was identified, half showed progression.[46] Clinically significant pain reduction of at least 2 points in NRS score was seen in 68% of patients at final follow-up, and mental and physical health scores also improved.[46] Select images from an MRgFUS ablation of desmoid fibromatosis are shown in **Fig. 2**.

Complications of MRgFUS were seen in 36% of patients, most commonly first or second degree skin burns, with the majority of these being mild; however, 7 patients required surgical debridement.[46] Most skin burns occurred early in the treatment experience, and decreased considerably as skin cooling techniques were introduced.[46] Transient nerve injury was seen in 21 treatments; in 2 additional cases nerve injury was present in patients who were lost to follow-up prior to resolution.[46] Thirty-five patients ultimately underwent another treatment modality due to progression of tumor or recurrent symptoms.[46]

Skin burn is the most common reported complication during MRgFUS of desmoid fibromatosis, but the risk can be decreased.[44] A minimum distance of 5 mm between the skin and tumor should be maintained, as well as and between the tumor and major neurovascular bundles.[44] Cutaneous scars should be avoided.[44] The near-field skin should be protected with a cool water bath overlying the transducer, and in some cases interposed gel pads or water bags.[47] In lesions such as in the extremities, the cumulative effect of large volume treatments can result in heating of the skin at the far field that is difficult to appreciate with MR thermometry and based on MR signal changes.[47] Water bags and gel pads should be placed on the far field skin for protection.[47] A fiberoptic temperature probe can also be placed on the far field skin for monitoring purposes.[47]

Given the variability of response to treatment, one study reviewed 13 treatments, evaluated a variety of technical factors which may contribute to success of the technique.[48] In this study, elongated sonications, which require significantly more energy, only resulted in 9% increase in ablation volume compared to short.[48] Utilizing these short sonications is likely safer for the skin and surrounding structures.[48] Optimization of an individual treatment plan may allow for better individual outcomes, though this needs further study.

Gadolinium-enhanced imaging is typically used to assess response of tumors to treatment; however, its administration precludes further treatment.[49] A mechanism of monitoring of ablated volume real time could provide valuable information and potentially improve outcomes. In a small study, intraprocedural rapid T2 mapping was evaluated and compared to post-treatment gadolinium-enhanced

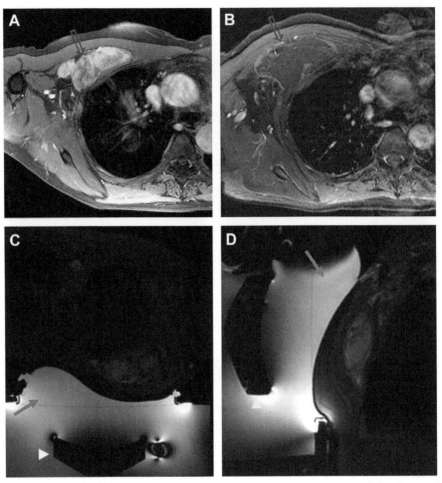

Fig. 2. Gadolinium-enhanced MR images show biopsy-proven desmoid fibromatosis of the chest wall (open *arrows*) from a diagnostic MRI examination prior to treatment (*A*) and immediately following (*B*) MRgFUS ablation. Note the peripheral rim of enhancement with non-enhancement of the majority of the tumor following treatment (*B*). Axial (*C*) and sagittal (*D*) T2 fat-saturated images obtained during the treatment show the patient lying supine over the ultrasound transducer (*arrowheads*). There is an interposed water bag (*arrows*) that conforms to the chest wall and protects the skin from burns.

images.[49] T2 values increased at the ablation site over the course of treatment, and areas with higher T2 value (mean 147.1 ms ± 18 ms) correlated well with non-perfused tumor.[49] In contrast, those of lower value on the T2 maps corresponded to areas of residual perfused tumor post-treatment, suggesting those areas may have benefitted from further treatment.[49]

ABDOMINAL WALL ENDOMETRIOSIS

Abdominal wall endometriosis is the presence of endometrial glands and stroma within the abdominal wall, resulting in characteristic cyclic abdominal pain with or without a palpable mass.[50] Open or laparoscopic resection is the typical management.[50]

Several publications have reported effective and safe treatment of abdominal wall endometriosis with ultrasound-guided HIFU.[51–54] In one such study, lesions were evaluated with MR imaging before and after treatment, and found MR imaging to be useful in identifying the location, its size, and post-ablation changes.[54] This information suggests that MRgFUS may be a valuable treatment modality for this indication; however, its use has not yet been described in the literature and research is needed.

PERIPHERAL NERVE ABLATION

Disruption of neural pathways may be utilized to treat neuropathic pain and/or spacticity.[8] Currently, this may be achieved by percutaneous RFA or surgically.[8] HIFU has been shown to be capable of causing both reversible and irreversible nerve conduction blocks in animal models and could become another option.[55–58]

A swine model aimed to ablate the intercostal nerve using MRgFUS, using the inferior margin of the rib as an anatomic landmark, and compared the results to ultrasound-guided RFA.[59] Both procedures produced lesions in the targeted intercostal nerve in 2 of 4 cases.[59]

Two swine studies evaluated the feasibility of using three-dimensional MR neurography to guide MRgFUS ablation of the sciatic nerve, and in one case a muscular branch, on a system integrated with a 3T scanner.[8,60] Both studies showed successful localization of the nerves with MR neurography, which were successfully ablated with a single sonication.[8] One of these studies assessed tractography, showing disruption after ablation.[60]

In human amputees, transected nerve endings were shown to be more sensitive to HIFU than intact nerves.[61] Further study on the role of MRgFUS in human peripheral nerves is needed. An ongoing clinical trial will assess MRgFUS of stump neuromas (ClinicalTrials.gov ID: NCT03255395).

VASCULAR MALFORMATIONS

First-line treatment of symptomatic low-flow vascular malformations is injection of a sclerosing agent, typically under ultrasound and/or fluoroscopic guidance.[62] In some situations, this may be challenging due to poor visualization with ultrasound or risk of injury to adjacent critical structures.[62] Complication rates range from 8% to 33%, with 20% being major in one study, including worsened pain, infection, skin necrosis, and nerve damage.[63,64] Percutaneous RF, laser, and cryoablation may be safe and effective alternatives, with good outcomes and lower complication rates (3.7% to 30%).[65–67] MRgFUS provides the added value of MR guidance, real-time thermal monitoring, and immediate evaluation of treatment success.[62]

HIFU has shown success in occluding small blood vessels; however, the effect can be temporary, with patency redemonstrated as early as 1 week.[68] Occlusion is thought to be secondary to thermal-induced coagulation of collagen in the vessel wall and endothelial damage leading to intraluminal thrombus.[68] Vessel rupture and subsequent hemorrhage have also been seen, particularly when tissue temperatures exceed 100°C.[68] In one ex vivo study, it was theorized that acoustic cavitation plays a role in HIFU-induced blood vessel rupture and can potentially be avoided by modulating HIFU intensity.[65]

One study retrospectively evaluated 5 patients who underwent MRgFUS treatment of low-flow intramuscular vascular malformations of the lower extremities.[62] The outpatient procedure was performed under general anesthesia.[62] Mean treatment time was 119 minutes, mean sonications 36, and mean energy 1967 J (658 to 3753), with the goal of achieving at least 60°C in the target tissue.[62] Patients were followed for 4 to 36 months, with a mean reduction in maximum and average pain of 81% and 75%, respectively.[62] The malformation volume decreased by a mean of 93%.[62] No complications were observed.[62] In another case report, a low-flow vascular malformation of the calf was successfully treated with MRgFUS.[69] The lesion reduced in size by greater than 30% at 3 month follow-up, and pain reduction was sustained for at least 13 months.[69]

SUMMARY

MRgFUS has a wide range of musculoskeletal applications. Some indications are well validated, specifically the treatment of painful osseous metastases and osteoid osteoma. Others are only beginning to be studied, such as the treatment of painful facet, SI and knee joints. MRgFUS of soft tissue lesions also shows promise, particularly in patients whom alternative modalities are not feasible or may result in significant morbidity, with the bulk of research focusing on desmoid fibromatosis. Ongoing and future research will illuminate the full potential for MRgFUS in the treatment of musculoskeletal conditions.

CLINICS CARE POINTS

- MRgFUS is safe and effective for the palliative treatment of painful bone metastases, with 77-79% response rates and 0.9-1.4% rate of major complication.

- MRgFUS has a 92.8% success rate in the treatment of osteoid osteoma with extremely low rates of adverse events.

- To be treatable by MRgFUS, the target lesion needs to be accessible by the beam path without intervening critical stuctures and greater than 1 cm from the skin.

DISCLOSURE

The author has nothing to disclose.

REFERENCES

1. Kawasaki M, Muramatsu S, Namba H, et al. Efficacy and safety of magnetic resonance-guided focused ultrasound treatment for refractory chronic pain of

medial knee osteoarthritis. Research Support, Non-U.S. Gov't. Int J Hyperthermia 2021;38(2):46–55.

2. di Biase L, Falato E, Caminiti ML, et al. Focused Ultrasound (FUS) for Chronic Pain Management: Approved and Potential Applications. Review. Neurol Res Int 2021;2021:8438498.

3. Coleman RE. Metastatic bone disease: clinical features, pathophysiology and treatment strategies. Review. Cancer Treat Rev 2001;27(3):165–76.

4. Baal JD, Chen WC, Baal U, et al. Efficacy and safety of magnetic resonance-guided focused ultrasound for the treatment of painful bone metastases: a systematic review and meta-analysis. Meta-Analysis Systematic Review. Skeletal Radiol 2021;50(12):2459–69.

5. Chow E, Hoskin P, Mitera G, et al. Update of the international consensus on palliative radiotherapy endpoints for future clinical trials in bone metastases. Research Support, Non-U.S. Gov't. Int J Radiat Oncol Biol Phys 2012;82(5):1730–7.

6. Han X, Huang R, Meng T, et al. The Roles of Magnetic Resonance-Guided Focused Ultrasound in Pain Relief in Patients With Bone Metastases: A Systemic Review and Meta-Analysis. Systematic Review. Front Times 2021;11:617295.

7. Dababou S, Marrocchio C, Scipione R, et al. High-Intensity Focused Ultrasound for Pain Management in Patients with Cancer. Review. Radiographics 2018;38(2):603–23.

8. Huisman M, van den Bosch MA, Wijlemans JW, et al. Effectiveness of reirradiation for painful bone metastases: a systematic review and meta-analysis. Meta-Analysis Review Systematic Review. Int J Radiat Oncol Biol Phys 2012;84(1):8–14.

9. Lee CC, Soon YY, Cheo T, et al. Stereotactic body radiation therapy versus conventional external beam radiation therapy for painful bone metastases: A systematic review and meta-analysis of randomized trials. Meta-Analysis Review Systematic Review. Crit Rev Oncol Hematol 2022;178:103775.

10. McDonald R, Chow E, Rowbottom L, et al. Incidence of pain flare in radiation treatment of bone metastases: A literature review. Review. J Bone Oncol 2014;3(3–4):84–9.

11. Liberman B, Gianfelice D, Inbar Y, et al. Pain palliation in patients with bone metastases using MR-guided focused ultrasound surgery: a multicenter study. Multicenter Study. Ann Surg Oncol 2009;16(1):140–6.

12. Napoli A, Anzidei M, Marincola BC, et al. Primary pain palliation and local tumor control in bone metastases treated with magnetic resonance-guided focused ultrasound. Clinical Trial. Invest Radiol. Jun 2013;48(6):351–8.

13. Zhou Q, Zhu XQ, Zhang J, et al. Changes in circulating immunosuppressive cytokine levels of cancer patients after high intensity focused ultrasound treatment. Clinical Trial Research Support, Non-U.S. Gov't. Ultrasound Med Biol 2008;34(1):81–7.

14. Huisman M, Lam MK, Bartels LW, et al. Feasibility of volumetric MRI-guided high intensity focused ultrasound (MR-HIFU) for painful bone metastases. J Ther Ultrasound 2014;2:16.

15. Tepelenis K, Skandalakis GP, Papathanakos G, et al. Osteoid Osteoma: An Updated Review of Epidemiology, Pathogenesis, Clinical Presentation, Radiological Features, and Treatment Option. Review. In Vivo 2021;35(4):1929–38.

16. Temple MJ, Waspe AC, Amaral JG, et al. Establishing a clinical service for the treatment of osteoid osteoma using magnetic resonance-guided focused ultrasound: overview and guidelines. Review. J Ther Ultrasound 2016;4:16.

17. Hu R, He P, Tian X, et al. Efficacy and safety of magnetic resonance-guided focused ultrasound for the treatment of osteoid osteoma: A systematic review and meta-analysis. Meta-Analysis Systematic Review. Eur J Radiol 2023;166:111006.

18. Masciocchi C, Zugaro L, Arrigoni F, et al. Radiofrequency ablation versus magnetic resonance guided focused ultrasound surgery for minimally invasive treatment of osteoid osteoma: a propensity score matching study. Randomized Controlled Trial. Eur Radiol 2016;26(8):2472–81.

19. Cobianchi Bellisari F, Palumbo P, Masciocchi C, et al. Needleless Ablation of Osteoid Osteoma and Osteoblastoma: The Emergent Role of MRgFUS. Review. J 2021;11(1):27.

20. Arrigoni F, Spiliopoulos S, de Cataldo C, et al. A Bicentric Propensity Score Matched Study Comparing Percutaneous Computed Tomography-Guided Radiofrequency Ablation to Magnetic Resonance-Guided Focused Ultrasound for the Treatment of Osteoid Osteoma. J Vasc Interv Radiol 2021;32(7):1044–51.

21. Geiger D, Napoli A, Conchiglia A, et al. MR-guided focused ultrasound (MRgFUS) ablation for the treatment of nonspinal osteoid osteoma: a prospective multicenter evaluation. Evaluation Study Multicenter Study Research Support, Non-U.S. Gov't. J Bone Joint Surg Am 2014;96(9):743–51.

22. Napoli A, Mastantuono M, Cavallo Marincola B, et al. Osteoid osteoma: MR-guided focused ultrasound for entirely noninvasive treatment. Radiology 2013;267(2):514–21.

23. Sharma KV, Yarmolenko PS, Celik H, et al. Comparison of Noninvasive High-Intensity Focused Ultrasound with Radiofrequency Ablation of Osteoid Osteoma. Clinical Trial Comparative Study Research Support, Non-U.S. Gov't. J Pediatr 2017;190:222–8.e1.

24. Arrigoni F, Bruno F, Palumbo P, et al. Magnetic resonance-guided focused ultrasound surgery treatment of non-spinal intra-articular osteoblastoma:

feasibility, safety, and outcomes in a single-center retrospective analysis. Int J Hyperthermia 2019; 36(1):768–75.

25. Izzo A, Zugaro L, Fascetti E, et al. Management of Osteoblastoma and Giant Osteoid Osteoma with Percutaneous Thermoablation Techniques. Review. J 2021;10(24):07.

26. de Cataldo C, Bruno F, Necozione S, et al. Weakening or Structural Strengthening? An Evaluation of Bone Density after MRgFUS Ablation for Treatment of Benign Bone Lesions. J Clin Med 2021; 11(1):29.

27. Arrigoni F, Lorenzo MG, Zugaro L, et al. MRgFUS in the treatment of MSK lesions: a review based on the experience of the University of L'Aquila, Italy. Transl Cancer Res 2014;3(5):442–8.

28. Arrigoni F, Barile A, Zugaro L, et al. Intra-articular benign bone lesions treated with Magnetic Resonance-guided Focused Ultrasound (MRgFUS): imaging follow-up and clinical results. Med Oncol 2017;34(4):55.

29. Van den Heuvel SAS, Cohen SPC, de Andres Ares J, et al. 3. Pain originating from the lumbar facet joints. Review. Pain Pract 2024;24(1):160–76.

30. Cohen SP, Bhaskar A, Bhatia A, et al. Consensus practice guidelines on interventions for lumbar facet joint pain from a multispecialty, international working group Research Support, Non-U.S. Gov't Research Support, U.S. Gov't, Non-P.H.S. . Reg Anesth Pain Med 2020;45(6):424–67.

31. Maas ET, Ostelo RW, Niemisto L, et al. Radiofrequency denervation for chronic low back pain. [Review]. Cochrane Database Syst Rev 2015;1(10): Cd008572.

32. Harnof S, Zibly Z, Shay L, et al. Magnetic resonance-guided focused ultrasound treatment of facet joint pain: summary of preclinical phase. J Ther Ultrasound 2014;2:9.

33. Aginsky R, LeBlang S, Hananel A, et al. Tolerability and Feasibility of X-ray Guided Non-Invasive Ablation of the Medial Branch Nerve with Focused Ultrasound: Preliminary Proof of Concept in a Pre-clinical Model. Research Support, Non-U.S. Gov't. Ultrasound Med Biol 2021;47(3):640–50.

34. Tiegs-Heiden CA, Hesley GK, Long Z, et al. MRI-guided focused ultrasound ablation of painful lumbar facet joints: a retrospective assessment of safety and tolerability in human subjects. Pain Med 2023; 24(11):1219–23.

35. Weeks EM, Platt MW, Gedroyc W. MRI-guided focused ultrasound (MRgFUS) to treat facet joint osteoarthritis low back pain–case series of an innovative new technique. Research Support, Non-U.S. Gov't. Eur Radiol 2012;22(12):2822–35.

36. Namba H, Kawasaki M, Izumi M, et al. Effects of MRgFUS Treatment on Musculoskeletal Pain: Comparison between Bone Metastasis and Chronic Knee/Lumbar Osteoarthritis. Clinical Trial Comparative Study. Pain Res Manag 2019;2019:4867904.

37. Perez J, Gofeld M, Leblang S, et al. Fluoroscopy-Guided High-Intensity Focused Ultrasound Neurotomy of the Lumbar Zygapophyseal Joints: A Clinical Pilot Study. Research Support, Non-U.S. Gov't. Pain Med 2022;23(1):67–75.

38. Simopoulos TT, Manchikanti L, Singh V, et al. A systematic evaluation of prevalence and diagnostic accuracy of sacroiliac joint interventions. Meta-Analysis Review Systematic Review. Pain Physician 2012;15(3):E305–44.

39. Cox RC, Fortin JD. The anatomy of the lateral branches of the sacral dorsal rami: implications for radiofrequency ablation. Pain Physician 2014;17(5):459–64.

40. Kaye EA, Maybody M, Monette S, et al. Ablation of the sacroiliac joint using MR-guided high intensity focused ultrasound: a preliminary experiment in a swine model. J Ther Ultrasound 2017;5:17.

41. Izumi M, Ikeuchi M, Kawasaki M, et al. MR-guided focused ultrasound for the novel and innovative management of osteoarthritic knee pain. Case Reports Validation Study. BMC Musculoskelet Disord 2013;14:267.

42. Prendergast K, Kryeziu S, Crago AM. The Evolving Management of Desmoid Fibromatosis. Review. Surg Clin North Am 2022;102(4):667–77.

43. Ghanouni P, Dobrotwir A, Bazzocchi A, et al. Magnetic resonance-guided focused ultrasound treatment of extra-abdominal desmoid tumors: a retrospective multicenter study. Multicenter Study. Eur Radiol 2017;27(2):732–40.

44. Griffin MO, Kulkarni NM, O'Connor SD, et al. Magnetic Resonance-Guided Focused Ultrasound: A Brief Review With Emphasis on the Treatment of Extra-abdominal Desmoid Tumors. Review. Ultrasound Q 2019;35(4):346–54.

45. Avedian RS, Bitton R, Gold G, et al. Is MR-guided High-intensity Focused Ultrasound a Feasible Treatment Modality for Desmoid Tumors? Research Support, N.I.H. Extramural. Clin Orthop 2016;474(3): 697–704.

46. Dux DM, Baal JD, Bitton R, et al. MR-guided focused ultrasound therapy of extra-abdominal desmoid tumors: a multicenter retrospective study of 105 patients. Eur Radiol 2023;24:24.

47. Bucknor MD, Rieke V. MRgFUS for desmoid tumors within the thigh: early clinical experiences. J Ther Ultrasound 2017;5:4.

48. Bucknor MD, Beroukhim G, Rieke V, et al. The impact of technical parameters on ablation volume during MR-guided focused ultrasound of desmoid tumors. Int J Hyperthermia 2019;36(1):473–6.

49. Morochnik S, Ozhinsky E, Rieke V, et al. T2-Mapping as a Predictor of Non-Perfused Volume in MRgFUS Treatment of Desmoid Tumors. Int J Hyperthermia 2019;36(1):1272–7.

50. Foley CE, Ayers PG, Lee TT. Abdominal Wall Endometriosis. Review. Obstet Gynecol Clin North Am 2022;49(2):369–80.

51. Xiao-Ying Z, Hua D, Jin-Juan W, et al. Clinical analysis of high-intensity focussed ultrasound ablation for abdominal wall endometriosis: a 4-year experience at a specialty gynecological institution. Research Support, Non-U.S. Gov't. Int J Hyperthermia 2019;36(1):87–94.

52. Shi S, Ni G, Ling L, et al. High-Intensity Focused Ultrasound in the Treatment of Abdominal Wall Endometriosis. Evaluation Study. J Minim Invasive Gynecol 2020;27(3):704–11.

53. Luo S, Zhang C, Huang JP, et al. Ultrasound-guided high-intensity focused ultrasound treatment for abdominal wall endometriosis: a retrospective study. Evaluation Study. Bjog 2017;124(Suppl 3):59–63.

54. Hu S, Liu Y, Chen R, et al. Exploring the Diagnostic Performance of Magnetic Resonance Imaging in Ultrasound-Guided High-Intensity Focused Ultrasound Ablation for Abdominal Wall Endometriosis. Front Physiol 2022;13:819259.

55. Colucci V, Strichartz G, Jolesz F, et al. Focused ultrasound effects on nerve action potential in vitro. Research Support, N.I.H., Extramural Research Support, Non-U.S. Gov't. Ultrasound Med Biol 2009;35(10):1737–47.

56. Foley JL, Little JW, Vaezy S. Image-guided high-intensity focused ultrasound for conduction block of peripheral nerves. Research Support, Non-U.S. Gov't Research Support, U.S. Gov't, Non-P.H.S. Ann Biomed Eng 2007;35(1):109–19.

57. Foley JL, Little JW, Vaezy S. Effects of high-intensity focused ultrasound on nerve conduction. Research Support, N.I.H., Extramural Research Support, Non-U.S. Gov't Research Support, U.S. Gov't, Non-P.H.S. Muscle Nerve 2008;37(2):241–50.

58. Foley JL, Little JW, Starr FL 3rd, et al. Image-guided HIFU neurolysis of peripheral nerves to treat spasticity and pain. Research Support, Non-U.S. Gov't Research Support, U.S. Gov't, Non-P.H.S. . Ultrasound Med Biol 2004;30(9):1199–207.

59. Gulati A, Loh J, Gutta NB, et al. Novel use of noninvasive high-intensity focused ultrasonography for intercostal nerve neurolysis in a swine model. Research Support, Non-U.S. Gov't. Reg Anesth Pain Med 2014;39(1):26–30.

60. Walker MR, Zhong J, Waspe AC, et al. Peripheral Nerve Focused Ultrasound Lesioning-Visualization and Assessment Using Diffusion Weighted Imaging. Front Neurol 2021;12:673060.

61. Mourad PD, Friedly JL, McClintic AM, et al. Intense Focused Ultrasound Preferentially Stimulates Transected Nerves Within Residual Limbs: Pilot Study. Research Support, Non-U.S. Gov't Research Support, U.S. Gov't, Non-P.H.S. Pain Med 2018;19(3):541–9.

62. Ghanouni P, Kishore S, Lungren MP, et al. Treatment of Low-Flow Vascular Malformations of the Extremities Using MR-Guided High Intensity Focused Ultrasound: Preliminary Experience. J Vasc Interv Radiol 2017;28(12):1739–44.

63. Ali S, Weiss CR, Sinha A, et al. The treatment of venous malformations with percutaneous sclerotherapy at a single academic medical center. Phlebology 2016;31(9):603–9.

64. Bowman J, Johnson J, McKusick M, et al. Outcomes of sclerotherapy and embolization for arteriovenous and venous malformations. Semin Vasc Surg 2013;26(1):48–54.

65. Hoerig CL, Serrone JC, Burgess MT, et al. Prediction and suppression of HIFU-induced vessel rupture using passive cavitation detection in an ex vivo model. J Ther Ultrasound 2014;2:14.

66. Augustine MR, Thompson SM, Powell GM, et al. Percutaneous MR Imaging-Guided Laser Ablation and Cryoablation for the Treatment of Pediatric and Adult Symptomatic Peripheral Soft Tissue Vascular Anomalies. J Vasc Interv Radiol 2021;32(10):1417–24.

67. Ge CX, Tai MZ, Chen T, et al. Analysis of 18 complex diffuse arteriovenous malformation cases treated with percutaneous radiofrequency ablation. Case Reports Research Support, Non-U.S. Gov't. BMC Cardiovasc Disord 2021;21(1):373.

68. Serrone J, Kocaeli H, Douglas Mast T, et al. The potential applications of high-intensity focused ultrasound (HIFU) in vascular neurosurgery. Review. J Clin Neurosci 2012;19(2):214–21.

69. van Breugel JM, Nijenhuis RJ, Ries MG, et al. Non-invasive magnetic resonance-guided high intensity focused ultrasound ablation of a vascular malformation in the lower extremity: a case report. J Ther Ultrasound 2015;3:23.

The Use of Focused Ultrasound Ablation for Movement Disorders

Nicole Silva, MD[a], Martin Green, BS[b], Daniel Roque, MD[c],
Vibhor Krishna, MD, SM[a],*

KEYWORDS

- Parkinson's disease • Focused ultrasound • Essential tremor • Ablation • Thalamotomy
- Pallidotomy

KEY POINTS

- Focused ultrasound ablation is a US Food and Drug Administration-approved treatment of medication-refractory essential tremor and Parkinson's disease.
- Research efforts are underway to optimize the ablation technique using advanced neuroimaging such as tractography.
- A multidisciplinary evaluation that discusses all the surgical options and highlights the pros and cons of each is required for informed decision-making in clinics.

INTRODUCTION

Ultrasounds are used in clinical neuroscience for transcranial and carotid dopplers and provide imaging guidance during neurosurgery. In recent history, the therapeutic applications of focused ultrasound made significant strides. Interestingly, the first description of therapeutic ultrasound dates back to the post-World War II era, when focused ultrasound ablation (FUSA) was used to treat 12 patients with Parkinson's disease (PD).[1] Dr Meyers and colleagues used atlas-based measurements, ventriculogram, and a stereotactic head frame to target the lentiform nucleus with a multibeam-focused ultrasound transducer (**Fig. 1**). However, FUSA did not gain wide traction because technological limitations prevented precise ultrasound targeting through the skull, and creating a thermal spot in the brain required craniotomy to provide a window.[2] These limitations were easily overcome using radiation, and therefore, stereotactic radiosurgery was rapidly established as an attractive treatment, while FUSA was abandoned without further testing and development.

Advances in ultrasound transducer technology and MR imaging have enabled reliable transcranial ultrasound delivery for FUSA, blood–brain barrier disruption (FUS BBBD), and neuromodulation. FUSA is Food and Drug Administration (FDA)-approved and insurance-reimbursed to treat essential tremor (ET), PD tremor, PD fluctuations, and PD dyskinesias. The therapeutic pipeline in the future looks promising for a variety of other neurologic disorders, such as epilepsy, neuropathic pain, and psychiatric illnesses. As the experience grows, FUSA is emerging as an excellent treatment option for patients with movement disorder who are at high risk for open surgery or who prefer to avoid hardware implantation. This article reviews the current literature and future directions of focused ultrasound to treat movement disorders.

[a] Department of Neurosurgery, University of North Carolina, 170 Manning Drive, Suite #2149, Chapel Hill, NC 27499, USA; [b] East Carolina University, School of Medicine; [c] UNC Movement Disorders Neuromodulation Program, Movement Disorders, Department of Neurology, University of North Carolina, 170 Manning Drive, Campus Box 7025, Chapel Hill, NC 27599, USA
* Corresponding author. 170 Manning Drive, Suite #2149, Chapel Hill, NC 27499.
E-mail address: vibhor_krishna@med.unc.edu
Twitter: @NicoleAASilva (N.S.)

Magn Reson Imaging Clin N Am 32 (2024) 651–659
https://doi.org/10.1016/j.mric.2024.04.003
1064-9689/24/© 2024 Elsevier Inc. All rights are reserved, including those for text and data mining, AI training, and similar technologies.

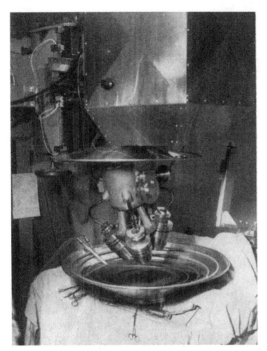

Fig. 1. Historical ultrasound transducer utilizing open craniotomy. (Journal Of Neurosurgery, January, 1959, 16, 1, Early Experiences With Ultrasonic Irradiation Of The Pallidofugal And Nigral Complexes In Hyperkinetic And Hypertonic Disorders, Meyers, 32-54. An Open Access or Creative Commons publishing model conveys no rights to use this material in any format without written permission from the JNS Publishing Group.)

ESSENTIAL TREMOR

ET is the most common movement disorder, affecting up to 1% of the global population, with a relatively equal distribution between men and women.[3] ET leads to functional disability[4] leading to social isolation and mental health consequences such as depression and anxiety.[5] Etiology is not definitively clear, but growing evidence points to aberrant, oscillatory activity within the cortico-olivo-cerebello-thalamic network.[6] When tremors become medication-refractory, some patients seek surgical intervention using deep brain stimulation or stereotactic radiofrequency thalamotomy, with the commercial availability of ventral intermediate nucleus (VIM) FUSA proving to catalyze a growing interest in the surgical management of tremors. FUSA was approved in 2016 by the FDA for unilateral treatment, and in 2022, it was approved to treat bilateral ET symptoms in a staged manner 9 months apart.

Unilateral Thalamotomy

The first single-center, open-label trial of VIM FUSA for ETs was completed in 2011, demonstrating

significant tremor reduction for up to 1 year.[7] It was followed by a multicenter, double-blinded, randomized controlled trial, in which patients assigned to VIM FUSA (n = 56) achieved a 47% reduction of hand tremor and 46% improvement in quality-of-life score compared to no tremor reduction in the sham cohort (n = 20).[8] These results were maintained in the 5 year follow-up, with continued reduction in hand tremors by up to 50%, emphasizing the durability of unilateral treatment of ET.[9] Following these landmark studies, other centers reported unblinded outcomes of open-label case series, reporting tremor reduction of greater than 40% and an increase in quality of life greater than 60%.[10–14] An interesting analysis by Yamatomo and colleagues[15] demonstrated that unilateral VIM FUSA improved ipsilateral axial and hand tremors in a small subgroup of patients with ET with severe tremors (n = 20). Finally, there has been limited literature on repeat ablation in the setting of suboptimal results, but one case report described a successful reablation, suggesting efficacy should a repeat FUSA be undertaken if tremor recurs.[16]

Bilateral Thalamotomy

Surgical ablation of bilateral basal ganglia and thalamic targets was documented with stereotactic radiofrequency ablation and was shown to result in substantial complications of ataxia, dysarthria, and dysphagia.[17] Therefore, bilateral VIM ablation was not offered secondary to a high risk of irreversible side effects.[18] After the success of unilateral VIM FUSA, there remained a clinical need to treat bilateral tremors, and the ability to accurately map real-time lesioning during FUSA created the ideal circumstances for exploring the safety of staged bilateral procedures. Martinez-Fernandez and colleagues were the first to describe a 67% to 81% improvement in clinical rating scale for tremor (CRST) scores in a case series.[19] This has been validated by a multicenter phase 2 trial, bilateral focused ultrasound thalamotomy for essential tremor (BEST-FUS), in which treating bilaterally increased quality of life and resulted in transient mild side effects in 7 of the 10 patients, characterized as ataxia and dysphagia.[20] Both studies evaluated patients for 3 months postoperatively; thus, further long-term effects are unknown. Another study retrospectively reviewed 5 patients who underwent bilateral VIM FUSA, yet at least 1 year apart between treatments, with encouraging results of decreased tremor and improved satisfaction with treatment.[21] There was one permanent adverse effect of dysarthria and discomfort of the tongue, yet the patient reported being satisfied with the treatment and further stated that they would repeat it despite the adverse effect. Finally, in a prospective, open-label trial of 11 patients who underwent VIM FUSA 1 year apart, there were only mild-to-moderate adverse effects, which included transient disequilibrium, and dysgeusia was the only adverse effect that persisted for about 3 months in 3 patients.[22] A large multicenter trial of staged bilateral VIM FUSA recently completed recruitment, and the results are expected to be published.

Optimization of Ventral Intermediate Nucleus Focused Ultrasound Ablation Technique

The research efforts to optimize the VIM FUSA technique involve standardizing the 3 treatment phases: targeting, subthreshold testing, and ablation. Tractography-based targeting was implemented to define 3 critical structures: the VIM, pyramidal tract, and medial lemniscus. These are linked to tremor relief, muscle weakness, and sensory loss, respectively (**Fig. 2**). The VIM was localized anterior to the sensory nucleus of the thalamus ventral caudal (VC), superior to the subthalamic white matter (approximated by the intercommissural plane), and medial to the pyramidal tracts.[23] Tractography-based VIM was localized slightly anteriorly and laterally compared to conventional imaging.[24] Early results indicate that accurate VIM visualization with patient-specific tractography may reduce the risk of adverse effects.[25–27] There is a need for further research to determine whether prospectively incorporating tractography can improve the safety and efficacy of VIM FUSA.

FUSA allows thermal neuromodulation for limited physiologic exploration paired with clinical testing (ie, subthreshold testing) before making the ablation permanent.[28] The optimal parameters for thermal neuromodulation for VIM FUSA were recently defined, and it was observed that using optimal parameters was associated with a reduced number of sonications, often required during subthreshold testing.[29] Further work is needed to refine the sonication parameters and determine associated improvements in clinical outcomes. Once the first ablation is delivered during VIM FUSA, the intraoperative tremor assessment becomes less reliable as real-time feedback to guide the need for further ablations because it tends to overestimate the long-term tremor relief.[26] Intraoperative tremor reduction reflects the combined effect of the ablated target (central core) and the surrounding tissue subjected to partial ablation and thermal neuromodulation (**Fig. 3**). Since the clinical effects of partial ablation and thermal neuromodulation can be partially reversed, intraoperative tremor assessment overestimates the long-term tremor relief. In one study, tremor improvement reduced from $68.1 \pm 15.5\%$ immediately following VIM FUSA to $56 \pm 13.2\%$ at 3 months postoperative.[26] While multiple ablative sonications are typically performed to achieve "sufficient" VIM ablation, each additional ablation carries a risk of developing side effects associated with the extension of the lesion beyond the VIM boundaries into the adjacent neural structures (**Fig. 4**). Therefore, further refinements in the FUSA technique are required to define whether "sufficient" ablation of the VIM target is achieved to provide long-term tremor relief without risking

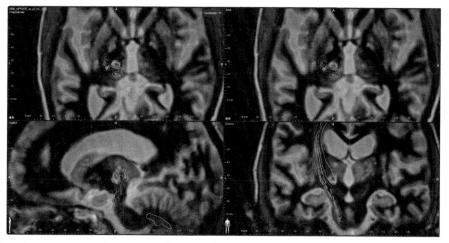

Fig. 2. Deterministic tractography to target the ventral intermediate nucleus (in *green*) for FUSA (lesion outlined in *orange*). The adjacent white matter tracts, including the internal capsule (*red*) and the medial lemniscus (*blue*), are shown.

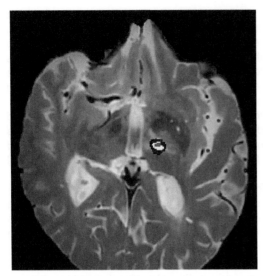

Fig. 3. Thermal neuromodulation in FUSA. During the ablation phase, the thermal spot comprises 3 distinct regions. The central core with ablated tissue (thermal dose ≥200 cumulative equivalent minutes [CEM]) is surrounded by a ring of partially ablated tissue receiving a thermal dose between 25 and 200 CEM. The thermal exposure of the outmost ring of tissue reaches the threshold for thermal neuromodulation. (*From* Sammartino et al. "Thermal Neuromodulation With Focused Ultrasound: Implications for the Technique of Subthreshold Testing". Neurosurgery. Sep 15 2021;89(4):610-616.)

side effects. One trial is currently testing whether ablating a predefined VIM volume (ie, ablating 70% of the VIM) is safe and efficacious (NCT#06331052).[30] This research will provide preliminary data for more extensive clinical trials testing the clinical utility of this approach.

PARKINSON'S DISEASE

PD is characterized by cardinal features of bradykinesia, rigidity, postural instability, and resting tremor.[31] Dopamine replacement can relieve motor symptoms, but patients eventually develop motor fluctuations with early wearing off or dyskinesias. Furthermore, tremor in Parkinson's has a much less reliable dopamine response than bradykinesia and rigidity.[32] Unilateral VIM FUSA was initially approved for tremor reduction in PD, while most recently, unilateral globus pallidus pars interna (GPi) FUSA received FDA approval for treating motor fluctuations and PD dyskinesias; presenting the option for patients to undergo this ablative procedure when these symptoms are most profound unilaterally and medically-refractory.

Unilateral Targets

One of the first published case reports of PD treatment by FUSA was a unilateral pallidotomy that was found to reduce tremor and dyskinesia by half.[33] The first randomized, controlled study for tremor-predominant PD was published in 2017, with a 62% decrease in tremor scores leading to the FDA approval of VIM FUSA for tremor-dominant PD.[34] The largest prospectively followed cohort to date of 48 patients with tremor-dominant PD who underwent thalamotomy demonstrated persistent tremor control for up to 2 years and with only mild side effects.[35] In 2019, Jung and colleagues[36] reported a 40% improvement in a dyskinesia-dominant PD cohort targeting unilateral posteroventral GPi. A larger phase-2 trial confirmed significant symptom improvement with excellent safety associated with GPI FUSA.[37] The phase-3

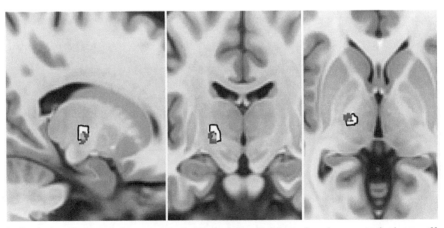

Fig. 4. Analyzing lesion characteristics associated with tremor relief (*green*) and unwanted adverse effects such as ataxia (*red*) relative to the ventral intermediate nucleus. (Sammartino et al. "Intraoperative lesion characterization after focused ultrasound thalamotomy" J Neurosurg. Dec 31 2021:1-9. An Open Access or Creative Commons publishing model conveys no rights to use this material in any format without written permission from the JNS Publishing Group.)

multicenter, prospective, blinded, randomized controlled trial of unilateral GPi FUSA found significantly more responders in the treatment arm than the sham group (70% vs 30%).[38] In the 12 month open-label follow-up, the symptom relief was durable. The most remarkable finding was the excellent safety profile of GPi FUSA.

Other research groups have focused on the subthalamic nucleus (STN) as a thermal ablation target. Martinez-Fernandez and colleagues demonstrated significant asymmetric tremor reduction (greater than 30%) with unilateral subthalamotomy in a pilot study of 10 patients with asymmetric parkinsonism.[39] This report was followed by a prospective, randomized, double-blind trial of subthalamotomy for those with significant asymmetric PD.[40] There was a significant decrease in motor impairment score by 10 points in those treated with STN FUSA compared to the control group, which showed a 1.7 point improvement.[40] Magara and colleagues[41] performed "pallidothalamic tractotomy" (PTT) in 13 patients and achieved up to 60% symptom relief. This treatment is currently being tested in a multicenter randomized trial.

Both unilateral subthalamotomy and pallidotomy thermal ablation have utility in the treatment of PD based on patient symptoms and treatment goals. The adverse effect profiles of both techniques differ due to anatomic locations. Pallidotomy adverse effects include hemiparesis secondary to thermal energy reaching the internal capsule, dysarthria, loss of taste, and less common, including ataxia.[33,41,42] Adverse effects noted after subthalamotomy included speech disturbance, dyskinesia, gait disequilibrium, and motor weakness noted to be localized to the face.[39,40]

Bilateral Targets

Studies for bilateral FUSA for PD are underway but are less numerous than those for ET. In one study, 15 patients underwent bilateral PTT thermal ablation, with up to 88% tremor relief, which was durable at 1 year follow-up.[42,43] Finally, another case report demonstrated successful symptom improvement in staged bilateral GPi FUSA.[44]

Other Therapeutic Parkinson's Disease Options

Other novel techniques are recently being explored for the treatment of PD, particularly neurodegeneration and dementia complications associated with the disease. One study utilized FUS BBBD to administer lysosomal enzyme glucocerebrosidase, shown in an animal model to slow neurodegeneration in PD, particularly in those carrying the GBA1 mutation, which is a gene that encodes the lysosomal enzyme glucocerebrosidase.[45]

Technique Optimization

Identifying and targeting the "hotspots" for optimal clinical improvement after FUSA for PD has been an important area of research. Specifically, GPi has proven to be a challenging target given its anatomy and surrounding white matter tracts. Sammartino and colleagues described 3 parcels within the GPi, which were determined by diffusion metric-based targeted segmentation. The posterior and central parcels proved to be the motor subregions and, thus, the optimal targets for FUSA for therapeutic effect in patients with PD.[46] GPi FUSA lesions were also localized to the posterior and central parcels, with 2 distinct "hotspots" for improvements in fluctuations and dyskinesias (**Fig. 5**). In summary, advanced neuroimaging can potentially optimize FUSA targeting to improve clinical outcomes in patients.

DYSTONIA AND OTHER RARE MOVEMENT DISORDERS

In comparison to PD and ET, dystonia has been a less well-studied movement disorder involving treatment with FUSA. There have been several case reports of patients with dystonia-type tremors, such as one associated with cervicobrachial dystonia, writer's cramp, and gene-associated tremor, who underwent VIM FUSA and achieved about 50% tremor reduction.[47] In another case report of musician's dystonia, a focal hand dystonia while playing an instrument, FUSA of the ventro-oral nucleus of the thalamus resulted in dramatic improvement of symptoms.[48] The same authors achieved similar outcomes in a cohort of 10 patients, of which durability of improvement in focal hand dystonia was noted up to 12 months after treatment.[49] There is now an open-label clinical trial recruiting focal hand dystonia patients for ventral-oral (Vo)-complex FUSA.[50] Finally, a rare neurodegenerative disease with limited options is X-linked dystonia-parkinsonism, which is found in male individuals with maternal ancestry from Panay Island, Philippines. A small case series of 3 patients were treated with unilateral PTT FUSA, with a 30% to 36% improvement of symptoms.[51]

FUTURE DIRECTIONS

There is a significant interest in studying brain network dynamics by comparing preoperative and postoperative conditions to determine the changes in dynamics associated with therapeutic intervention. However, these investigations were

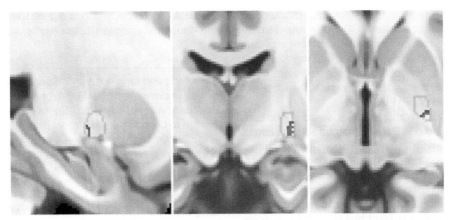

Fig. 5. "Hot spot" location for highest therapeutic effect after FUSA, the posterior parcel of GPi. Two distinct locations were found to be associated with the improvement in motor fluctuations (*blue*) and dyskinesias (*red*). (Sammartino et al. "Intraoperative lesion characterization after focused ultrasound thalamotomy" J Neurosurg. Dec 31 2021:1-9. An Open Access or Creative Commons publishing model conveys no rights to use this material in any format without written permission from the JNS Publishing Group.)

often limited by safety concerns associated with neuroimaging acquisition with implanted intracranial hardware. FUSA affords a unique opportunity to investigate brain network dynamics given the lack of implantable devices, allowing for extensive studies to develop a deeper understanding of the neuromodulatory effect of therapy. One goal of connectomics research is to uncover the FUSA mechanisms of action to inform the future development of treatments for neurologic and psychiatric conditions. Magnetoencephalography was utilized to study mu rhythm—an established neurophysiologic correlate of movement—and found VIM FUSA resulted in a reduction of mu rhythm, leading to postulations that ablation improved synchronization of the motor cortex via thalamocortical circuits.[52] In another study, the authors used functional near-infrared spectroscopy to analyze hemodynamic changes in the cerebral cortex, identifying specific cortical activity changes after VIM FUSA, further providing evidence that there are changes in neural networks posttreatment.[53] Resting-state functional MR imaging has also been used to study the changes of neural networks, and several studies have found that VIM FUSA modulated functional connectivity in the cerebello-thalamo-cortical tremor network in addition to the visual processing areas and superior temporal gyrus.[54,55]

Interdisciplinary Approaches to Offering Focused Ultrasound Ablation to Treat Movement Disorders

Much literature is evident on the overarching values afforded by multidisciplinary and interdisciplinary management of neurologic disorders, with a series of publications available for numerous movement disorders, including Parkinsonian syndromes, Huntington's disease, and hereditary ataxias.[56–59] Though distinctions have not been formally compared in published works, a review of available literature and marketing for multidisciplinary versus interdisciplinary clinics would suggest that the fundamental difference between the two formats is in the immediacy of communication and, thus, comprehensive evaluation by multiple team members.[60] As multidisciplinary teams may render services in different physical locations on separate dates, this model is more easily reproduced when servicing large patient populations across multiple organizations. Developing and maintaining an interdisciplinary approach demands greater coordination between providers and other essential team members to ensure availability but with the benefits of subsequent, live discussion among team members who can agree on the best diagnostic and therapeutic pathways for the patients they evaluate.

The introduction of FUSA into clinical care of neurologic conditions has proven attractive for patients to seek evaluation for treatment when previously they were less likely to consider alternative surgical techniques.[61] However, so many of the treatable disorders have symptoms that are inherently heterogeneous between patients and even with an overlap of treatable symptoms between disorders. This is best highlighted by tremor, a symptom that exists across multiple primary movement disorders and has garnered a multiaxis classification schema to help better distinguish phenomenology and etiology when evaluating a patient.[62] The risks of misclassifying tremor can include suboptimal FUSA results and increased risk of procedural complications. The value of a multidisciplinary or interdisciplinary team approach for FUSA could thus be in a more accurate assessment of the patient's presurgical neurologic function as well as a personalized series of surgical expectations offered by multiple potential team members: a movement disorders specialist for diagnostic accuracy, a neurosurgeon for surgical appropriateness, physical therapist for formal balance assessment, and occupational therapist for objective measures related to intrusive movements disorders affecting the upper limb function. However, publications on the specific role and construct of these clinics are imminently needed to help guide organizations toward a clinically useful standard of care that will yield optimized outcomes for patients with movement disorders.

SUMMARY

The current literature and outcomes reported from FUSA for treating movement disorders are encouraging. FUSA provides an alternative treatment to patients unable to or unwilling to undergo deep brain stimulation (DBS). As neuroimaging and FUS technology advance, we expect further improvement in treatment outcomes. With more real-world data, the longevity of this treatment's outcomes will become clear. A multidisciplinary approach to treating patients with movement disorder is required for diagnostic accuracy, surgical appropriateness, and risk assessment, highlighting all available treatment options while carefully weighing the risks and benefits in each clinical scenario.

CLINICS CARE POINTS

- Focused Ultrasound ablation is a non-invasive surgical option for treatment of Essential Tremor and Parkinson's disease, proving to be a therapeutic option for those who are poor surgical candidates or do not want to undergo invasive surgery.

- Focused ultrasound ablation research is rapidly advancing, and outcomes of patients treated by this novel technique are proving to be quite successful.

DISCLOSURES

Dr V. Krishna is funded by NIH, United States. All other authors do not have commercial or financial conflicts of interest, and there are no funding sources for all authors.

REFERENCES

1. Fry WJ, Mosberg WH Jr, Barnard JW, et al. Production of focal destructive lesions in the central nervous system with ultrasound. J Neurosurg 1954; 11(5):471–8.
2. Meyers R, Fry WJ, Fry FJ, et al. Early experiences with ultrasonic irradiation of the pallidofugal and nigral complexes in hyperkinetic and hypertonic disorders. J Neurosurg 1959;16(1):32–54.
3. Haubenberger D, Hallett M. Essential Tremor. N Engl J Med 2018;378(19):1802–10.
4. Louis ED, Barnes L, Albert SM, et al. Correlates of functional disability in essential tremor. Mov Disord 2001;16(5):914–20.
5. Woods SP, Scott JC, Fields JA, et al. Executive dysfunction and neuropsychiatric symptoms predict lower health status in essential tremor. Cognit Behav Neurol 2008;21(1):28–33.
6. Schnitzler A, Munks C, Butz M, et al. Synchronized brain network associated with essential tremor as revealed by magnetoencephalography. Mov Disord 2009;24(11):1629–35.
7. Elias WJ, Huss D, Voss T, et al. A pilot study of focused ultrasound thalamotomy for essential tremor. N Engl J Med 2013;369(7):640–8.
8. Elias WJ, Lipsman N, Ondo WG, et al. A Randomized Trial of Focused Ultrasound Thalamotomy for Essential Tremor. N Engl J Med 2016;375(8):730–9.
9. Cosgrove GR, Lipsman N, Lozano AM, et al. Magnetic resonance imaging-guided focused ultrasound thalamotomy for essential tremor: 5-year follow-up results. J Neurosurg 2023;138(4):1028–33.
10. Abe K, Horisawa S, Yamaguchi T, et al. Focused Ultrasound Thalamotomy for Refractory Essential Tremor: A Japanese Multicenter Single-Arm Study. Neurosurgery 2021;88(4):751–7.
11. Park YS, Jung NY, Na YC, et al. Four-year follow-up results of magnetic resonance-guided focused ultrasound thalamotomy for essential tremor. Mov Disord 2019;34(5):727–34.
12. Sinai A, Nassar M, Eran A, et al. Magnetic resonance-guided focused ultrasound thalamotomy for essential tremor: a 5-year single-center experience. J Neurosurg 2019;133:1–8.
13. Halpern CH, Santini V, Lipsman N, et al. Three-year follow-up of prospective trial of focused ultrasound thalamotomy for essential tremor. Neurology 2019; 93(24):e2284–93.
14. Lipsman N, Schwartz ML, Huang Y, et al. MR-guided focused ultrasound thalamotomy for essential tremor: a proof-of-concept study. Lancet Neurol 2013;12(5):462–8.
15. Yamamoto K, Sarica C, Elias GJB, et al. Ipsilateral and axial tremor response to focused ultrasound thalamotomy for essential tremor: clinical outcomes and probabilistic mapping. J Neurol Neurosurg

Psychiatry 2022. https://doi.org/10.1136/jnnp-2021-328459.

16. Weidman EK, Kaplitt MG, Strybing K, et al. Repeat magnetic resonance imaging-guided focused ultrasound thalamotomy for recurrent essential tremor: case report and review of MRI findings. J Neurosurg 2019;25:1–6.

17. Alomar S, King NK, Tam J, et al. Speech and language adverse effects after thalamotomy and deep brain stimulation in patients with movement disorders: A meta-analysis. Mov Disord 2017;32(1):53–63.

18. Alshaikh J, Fishman PS. Revisiting bilateral thalamotomy for tremor. Clin Neurol Neurosurg 2017;158:103–7.

19. Martinez-Fernandez R, Mahendran S, Pineda-Pardo JA, et al. Bilateral staged magnetic resonance-guided focused ultrasound thalamotomy for the treatment of essential tremor: a case series study. J Neurol Neurosurg Psychiatry 2021;92(9):927–31.

20. Iorio-Morin C, Yamamoto K, Sarica C, et al. Bilateral Focused Ultrasound Thalamotomy for Essential Tremor (BEST-FUS Phase 2 Trial). Mov Disord 2021; 36(11):2653–62.

21. Fukutome K, Hirabayashi H, Osakada Y, et al. Bilateral Magnetic Resonance Imaging-Guided Focused Ultrasound Thalamotomy for Essential Tremor. Stereotact Funct Neurosurg 2022;100(1):44–52.

22. Scantlebury N, Rohringer CR, Rabin JS, et al. Safety of Bilateral Staged Magnetic Resonance-Guided Focused Ultrasound Thalamotomy for Essential Tremor. Mov Disord Clin Pract 2023;10(10):1559–61.

23. Sammartino F, Krishna V, King NK, et al. Tractography-Based Ventral Intermediate Nucleus Targeting: Novel Methodology and Intraoperative Validation. Mov Disord 2016;31(8):1217–25.

24. Boutet A, Ranjan M, Zhong J, et al. Focused ultrasound thalamotomy location determines clinical benefits in patients with essential tremor. Brain 2018;141(12):3405–14.

25. Lehman VT, Lee KH, Klassen BT, et al. MRI and tractography techniques to localize the ventral intermediate nucleus and dentatorubrothalamic tract for deep brain stimulation and MR-guided focused ultrasound: a narrative review and update. Neurosurg Focus 2020;49(1):E8. https://doi.org/10.3171/2020.4.FOCUS20170.

26. Krishna V, Sammartino F, Agrawal P, et al. Prospective Tractography-Based Targeting for Improved Safety of Focused Ultrasound Thalamotomy. Neurosurgery 2019;84(1):160–8.

27. Agrawal M, Garg K, Samala R, et al. Outcome and Complications of MR Guided Focused Ultrasound for Essential Tremor: A Systematic Review and Meta-Analysis. Front Neurol 2021;12:654711. https://doi.org/10.3389/fneur.2021.654711.

28. Krishna V, Sammartino F, Rezai A. A Review of the Current Therapies, Challenges, and Future Directions of Transcranial Focused Ultrasound Technology: Advances in Diagnosis and Treatment. JAMA Neurol 2018;75(2):246–54.

29. Sammartino F, Snell J, Eames M, et al. Thermal Neuromodulation With Focused Ultrasound: Implications for the Technique of Subthreshold Testing. Neurosurgery 2021;89(4):610–6.

30. Sammartino F, Yeh FC, Krishna V. Intraoperative lesion characterization after focused ultrasound thalamotomy. J Neurosurg 2021;1–9. https://doi.org/10.3171/2021.10.JNS211651.

31. Postuma RB, Berg D, Stern M, et al. MDS clinical diagnostic criteria for Parkinson's disease. Mov Disord 2015;30(12):1591–601.

32. Zach H, Dirkx MF, Roth D, et al. Dopamine-responsive and dopamine-resistant resting tremor in Parkinson disease. Neurology 2020;95(11):e1461–70.

33. Na YC, Chang WS, Jung HH, et al. Unilateral magnetic resonance-guided focused ultrasound pallidotomy for Parkinson disease. Neurology 2015; 85(6):549–51.

34. Bond AE, Shah BB, Huss DS, et al. Safety and Efficacy of Focused Ultrasound Thalamotomy for Patients With Medication-Refractory, Tremor-Dominant Parkinson Disease: A Randomized Clinical Trial. JAMA Neurol 2017;74(12):1412–8.

35. Chua MMJ, Blitz SE, Ng PR, et al. Focused Ultrasound Thalamotomy for Tremor in Parkinson's Disease: Outcomes in a Large, Prospective Cohort. Mov Disord 2023;38(10):1962–7.

36. Jung NY, Park CK, Kim M, et al. The efficacy and limits of magnetic resonance-guided focused ultrasound pallidotomy for Parkinson's disease: a Phase I clinical trial. J Neurosurg 2018;1–9. https://doi.org/10.3171/2018.2.JNS172514.

37. Eisenberg HM, Krishna V, Elias WJ, et al. MR-guided focused ultrasound pallidotomy for Parkinson's disease: safety and feasibility. J Neurosurg 2020; 135(3):792–8.

38. Krishna V, Fishman PS, Eisenberg HM, et al. Trial of Globus Pallidus Focused Ultrasound Ablation in Parkinson's Disease. N Engl J Med 2023;388(8):683–93.

39. Martinez-Fernandez R, Rodriguez-Rojas R, Del Alamo M, et al. Focused ultrasound subthalamotomy in patients with asymmetric Parkinson's disease: a pilot study. Lancet Neurol 2018;17(1):54–63.

40. Martinez-Fernandez R, Manez-Miro JU, Rodriguez-Rojas R, et al. Randomized Trial of Focused Ultrasound Subthalamotomy for Parkinson's Disease. N Engl J Med 2020;383(26):2501–13.

41. Magara A, Buhler R, Moser D, et al. First experience with MR-guided focused ultrasound in the treatment of Parkinson's disease. J Ther Ultrasound 2014;2:11.

42. Gallay MN, Moser D, Rossi F, et al. MRgFUS Pallidothalamic Tractotomy for Chronic Therapy-Resistant Parkinson's Disease in 51 Consecutive Patients: Single Center Experience. Front Surg 2019;6:76.

43. Gallay MN, Moser D, Magara AE, et al. Bilateral MR-Guided Focused Ultrasound Pallidothalamic Tractotomy for Parkinson's Disease With 1-Year Follow-Up. Front Neurol 2021;12:601153. https://doi.org/10.3389/fneur.2021.601153.

44. Stieglitz LH, Mahendran S, Oertel MF, et al. Bilateral Focused Ultrasound Pallidotomy for Parkinson-Related Facial Dyskinesia-A Case Report. Mov Disord Clin Pract 2022;9(5):647–51.

45. Meng Y, Pople CB, Huang Y, et al. Putaminal Recombinant Glucocerebrosidase Delivery with Magnetic Resonance-Guided Focused Ultrasound in Parkinson's Disease: A Phase I Study. Mov Disord 2022;37(10):2134–9.

46. Sammartino F, Marsh R, Yeh FC, et al. Radiological identification of the globus pallidus motor subregion in Parkinson's disease. J Neurosurg 2021;1–9. https://doi.org/10.3171/2021.7.JNS21858.

47. Fasano A, Llinas M, Munhoz RP, et al. MRI-guided focused ultrasound thalamotomy in non-ET tremor syndromes. Neurology 2017;89(8):771–5.

48. Horisawa S, Yamaguchi T, Abe K, et al. A single case of MRI-guided focused ultrasound ventro-oral thalamotomy for musician's dystonia. J Neurosurg 2018;131(2):384–6.

49. Horisawa S, Yamaguchi T, Abe K, et al. Magnetic Resonance-Guided Focused Ultrasound Thalamotomy for Focal Hand Dystonia: A Pilot Study. Mov Disord 2021;36(8):1955–9.

50. Maamary J, Peters J, Kyle K, et al. Evaluation of the efficacy and safety of MRI-guided focused ultrasound (MRgFUS) for focal hand dystonia: study protocol for an open-label non-randomised clinical trial. BMJ Neurol Open 2023;5(2):e000522. https://doi.org/10.1136/bmjno-2023-000522.

51. Jamora RDG, Chang WC, Taira T. Transcranial Magnetic Resonance-Guided Focused Ultrasound in X-Linked Dystonia-Parkinsonism. Life 2021;11(5). https://doi.org/10.3390/life11050392.

52. Chang JW, Min BK, Kim BS, et al. Neurophysiologic correlates of sonication treatment in patients with essential tremor. Ultrasound Med Biol 2015;41(1):124–31.

53. Gurgone S, De Salvo S, Bonanno L, et al. Changes in cerebral cortex activity during a simple motor task after MRgFUS treatment in patients affected by essential tremor and Parkinson's disease: a pilot study using functional NIRS. Phys Med Biol 2023. https://doi.org/10.1088/1361-6560/ad164e.

54. Kindler C, Upadhyay N, Purrer V, et al. MRgFUS of the nucleus ventralis intermedius in essential tremor modulates functional connectivity within the classical tremor network and beyond. Parkinsonism Relat Disorders 2023;115:105845. https://doi.org/10.1016/j.parkreldis.2023.105845.

55. Dahmani L, Bai Y, Li M, et al. Focused ultrasound thalamotomy for tremor treatment impacts the cerebello-thalamo-cortical network. NPJ Parkinsons Dis 2023;9(1):90.

56. Qamar MA, Harington G, Trump S, et al. Multidisciplinary Care in Parkinson's Disease. Int Rev Neurobiol 2017;132:511–23.

57. Lidstone SC, Bayley M, Lang AE. The evidence for multidisciplinary care in Parkinson's disease. Expert Rev Neurother 2020;20(6):539–49.

58. Cruickshank TM, Reyes AP, Penailillo LE, et al. Effects of multidisciplinary therapy on physical function in Huntington's disease. Acta Neurol Scand 2018;138(6):500–7.

59. Thompson JA, Cruickshank TM, Penailillo LE, et al. The effects of multidisciplinary rehabilitation in patients with early-to-middle-stage Huntington's disease: a pilot study. Eur J Neurol 2013;20(9):1325–9.

60. Saxena N, Rizk DV. The interdisciplinary team: the whole is larger than the parts. Adv Chron Kidney Dis 2014;21(4):333–7.

61. Hopfner F, Deuschl G. Managing Essential Tremor. Neurotherapeutics 2020;17(4):1603–21.

62. Bhatia KP, Bain P, Bajaj N, et al. Consensus Statement on the classification of tremors. from the task force on tremor of the International Parkinson and Movement Disorder Society. Mov Disord 2018;33(1):75–87.

MR-guided Focused Ultrasound Thalamotomy for Chronic Pain

Marco Colasurdo, MD[a], Abdul-Kareem Ahmed, MD[b],
Dheeraj Gandhi, MD, FACR[b,c,d,e,f,*]

KEYWORDS

- Chronic neuropathic pain • Advanced MR imaging • Pain • Focused ultrasound • Thalamotomy

KEY POINTS

- We provide an overview of the principal anatomic pathways of pain, highlighting functional aspects of chronic pain.
- We summarize the current available literature on MR-guided focused ultrasound thalamotomy in chronic neuropathic pain.
- We describe technical challenges related to cerebral thermoablation.
- We also provide an overview of ongoing trials that will elucidate further evidence in the near future.

HISTORICAL BACKGROUND

The International Association for the Study of Pain defines chronic pain as "persistent or recurrent pain lasting longer than 3 months,"[1] whereas neuropathic pain is usually defined as "pain caused by a lesion or disease of the somatosensory nervous system."[2] Chronic neuropathic pain (CNP) is a highly prevalent disorder, with an estimated prevalence of about 8%, and significant associated morbidity.[3] Patients facing CNP have often reached a point where the pain networks will no longer provide a protection and healing mechanism, letting pain become a disease of its own.[4] Thus, culminating in alteration of the experience of pain perception with changes in the biochemistry of pain transduction.[5]

Nociception in humans has historically been believed to be homed in 3 essential areas: the primary somatosensory area, the thalamus, and the anterior cingulate cortex (ACC). Despite these preconceptions, the strong influence of functional MR (fMR) imaging and PET studies has brought to light how pain, the fifth vital sign, entails a much more complex integration and modulation, both of which occur throughout numerous brain and medullary structures with major pathways across the opercular–insular cortex and thalamic nuclei. In CNP, these areas are abnormally recruited, often bilaterally, and surprisingly also in response to below-threshold stimuli.[6]

Therefore, it does not come as a surprise that the recommendation of the National Institute for Health and Clinical Excellence for first-line and second-line treatment options for CNP suggests the use of antidepressants and antiepileptic drugs.[7] Third-line treatments include the use of opioids alone or combined with first-line and

[a] Department of Interventional Radiology, Oregon Health and Science University, Portland, OR 97239, USA; [b] Department of Neurosurgery, University of Maryland School of Medicine; [c] Division of Neurointerventional Surgery, Department of Diagnostic Radiology, University of Maryland School of Medicine, University of Maryland, 22 South Green Street, Baltimore, MD 21201, USA; [d] Department of Radiology, University of Maryland School of Medicine, 22 South Green Street, Baltimore, MD 21201, USA; [e] Department of Neurology, University of Maryland School of Medicine, 22 South Green Street, Baltimore, MD 21201, USA; [f] Department of Neurosurgery, University of Maryland School of Medicine, 22 South Green Street, Baltimore, MD 21201, USA
* Corresponding author. Division of Neurointerventional Surgery, Department of Diagnostic Radiology, University of Maryland School of Medicine, 22 South Green Street, Baltimore, MD 21201.
E-mail address: dgandhi@umm.edu

Magn Reson Imaging Clin N Am 32 (2024) 661–672
https://doi.org/10.1016/j.mric.2024.04.005
1064-9689/24/© 2024 Elsevier Inc. All rights reserved, including those for text and data mining, AI training, and similar technologies.

second-line agents. However, single-agent therapies often fail, and patients develop medically resistant CNP seeking nonpharmacological approaches. Neuromodulation, specifically spinal cord stimulation, is one of the possible intervention options available to these patients. It received FDA approval in 1989 and, since then, has greatly contributed to improving outcomes despite a higher rate of long-term complications.[8,9]

The complexity and higher chance for complications during open surgical interventions at the level of the brainstem quickly shifted the interest to stereotactic ablation procedures. The experience with stereotactic radiosurgical ablation of thalamic nuclei[10,11] unveiled the role of this structure as the primary target. However, these interventions often cause somatosensory deficits and have shown limited clinical use, witnessed by scarce literature moreover with controversial long-term results.[12] The placement of deep brain stimulation electrodes is one of the potential alternatives. It was first pioneered for the treatment of Parkinson's disease (PD) and has been the subject of investigations in patients with CNP. Despite the potential advantage of reversibility, there were 2 open-label trials, which were terminated early due to limited efficacy.[13] Thus, the use of deep brain stimulation in CNP remains off-label in the United States. MR-guided focused ultrasound (MRgFUS) has emerged as a promising alternative with an increasing number of active clinical trials, not limited to CNP but also including patients with essential tremor, PD, trigeminal neuralgia (TN), and so on.

In this article, we provide an overview of the major anatomic pain pathways and summarize the current knowledge about MRgFUS regarding chronic neuropathic pain highlighting risks, benefits, and future directions.

THE "FUNCTIONAL" ANATOMY OF PAIN

Today, it would be hard to imagine pain being anything but a conscious sensation while not long ago, pain integration in the central nervous system was believed to be confined to subcortical structures and mostly centered in the thalamus. Subsequent advances in knowledge showed how the experience of pain was built through a much more complex interaction between sensory, cognitive, and affective dimensions with extensive involvement of supraspinal structures in pain management and modulation.[14] In 1991, Jones and colleagues[15] published the first study demonstrating activations in multiple cortical and subcortical regions during painful stimuli in normal subjects. Since then, many investigators have assessed brain responses to pain through PET, fMR imaging, and arterial spin labeling (ASL), with functional activation of regions secondary to increases in regional cerebral blood flow in PET and ASL and by subtle changes of blood oxygen level-dependent signal in fMR imaging.[16–18]

A few years later, Melzack's neuromatrix replaced the gate theory and citing his words: *"The anatomical substrate of the body-self, I propose, is a large, widespread network of neurons that consists of loops between the thalamus and cortex as well as between the cortex and limbic system. I have labeled the entire network, whose spatial distribution and synaptic links are initially determined genetically and later are sculpted by sensory inputs, as a neuromatrix."*[19] In the neuromatrix, the primary and secondary somatosensory cortices, the lateral thalamic nuclei, and the posterior insula constitute the lateral pain system; the dorsal anterior cingulate cortex (dACC), the amygdala, the anterior insula, and the medial thalamic nuclei form the medial pain system. In addition, a functional descending pain system includes the dACC, the prefrontal cortex (PFC), and the periaqueductal gray matter, with dense functional connections via the thalamus.[20]

Activation of the lateral system is believed to relay discriminative information regarding the location, duration, and intensity of painful stimuli. The primary somatosensory area, located just across the postcentral gyrus, has been known to harbor somatotopy for painful and nonpainful stimuli,[21] while the secondary somatosensory area, located in the parietal operculum, lacking a specific somatotopic organization, has shown activation with intensities that follow noxious stimuli.[22] Both somatosensory cortical areas likely receive simultaneous, bilateral stimuli, short-circuiting multiple cortico-cortical, transcallosal, and thalamic anastomosis, shortening processing times of noxious activations[23,24] consistent with the notion that it would be impossible to define the boundaries of the somatosensory system. Cognitive processing of pain has been associated with activations in the rostral or dorsal ACC.[25] While affective, empathic, and emotional responses to pain provoke intense activations in the posterior insula and rostral/dorsal ACC,[26] the only known cortical region in which direct stimulation induces physical pain is the posterior operculo-insular cortex.[27] In addition, functional connectivity studies have shown how painful stimulation itself can induce a decrease in the activation of several core structures of the default mode network (DMN).[28]

The thalamus plays a central role within the complex connections of the pain network, harboring several functional pathways of the pain neuromatrix. Ascending fibers from the spinal cord, spinothalamic tracts, project to specific thalamic nuclei through the brainstem; each nucleus will then have different projections and interconnections with cortical structures following a precise, organized, hierarchy. Most projections to the primary and secondary somatosensory cortices originate from the ventral posterior medial (VPM) and ventral posterior lateral (VPL) nuclei.[29] The mediodorsal (MD) thalamic nucleus demonstrates dense interconnections with the PFC, the medial temporal regions, the cerebellum, and numerous subcortical structures and has an essential role in managing activities related to cognition and emotion.[30,31] Similarly to the MD, the medial pulvinar nucleus (PuM) has shown the most significant overlap of projections with the 6 major brain cortical areas.[32] Lesions in either the PuM or the MD have historically shown pain relief, however, with limited lasting effects.[33] Finally, the centrum medianum (CM) and central lateral (CL) nuclei demonstrate reciprocal connections with the affective pain processing pathways with projections to the ACC and PFC. While the CM also participates in sensorimotor coordination, the CL nucleus exhibits connections with areas mediating both affective, cognitive, and discriminative components of pain, making it an exquisite surgical target of choice among thalamic nuclei.[34] In addition, the CL nucleus and, in particular, its most posterior extension central lteral posterior (CLp), only observed in nonhuman primates and humans, seem to have gradually lost its normal function with time and can sustain and amplify overproduction of low frequencies. This process has been defined as thalamocortical dysrhythmia,[35–37] a mechanism demonstrated by quantitative electroencephalography.[37,38] Interestingly, selective targeting of this nucleus can restore normal thalamocortical dynamics while preserving functions supported by other structures.[35] Moreover, while the connectivity patterns of VPL and VPM are spatially limited, the CL nucleus has multiple interactions with motor, cognitive, and alerting aspects of pain.[39,40]

CNP has been shown to alter cortical dynamics in pain processing with much more prominent activations involving regions entrusted with processing of cognitive and emotional aspects of noxious stimuli.[41] Prolonged stimulations, such as those experienced by patients with CNP can lead to disorganized neuroplastic changes at the cortical level, involving the DMN (**Fig. 1**), leading to sensitization,[42] with the most common reorganization consisting of dissociation of the DMN, and increased association between the medial PFC and the insula. Interestingly, the extent of the reorganization seems to be a function of the intensity and the duration of the painful stimulus.[43] Future studies are needed to further investigate the role of neuroplasticity for the treatment of neuropathic pain syndromes.

MR-guided Focused Ultrasound

The ability to propagate ultrasound waves through the human skull in order to deliver precise amounts of energy to restricted areas of the brain is nowadays well established, although not very well known among all specialties. Fry and colleagues[44–46] and Lele[47] with animals and subsequently with early clinical studies showed how ultrasound waves could be focused into a beam and directed through a piece of skull to induce lesions in animal brains immersed in water.

Among the numerous technical challenges behind the delivery of ultrasound-generated energy to deep brain structures, skull thickness[48] has represented the most complicated to overcome. Ultrasound waves transmission to intracranial structures is deeply affected by structural characteristics of the skull,[49] and while acoustic windows can vary greatly among different patients based on age, sex, bone thickness, presence of spiculae, and other factors,[50] ultimately ultrasound monitoring of intracranial arteries blood flow through the temporal bone can be easily achieved using the Doppler effect.[51]

Physics has shown us how acoustic waves can be attenuated 30–60 times more in bone when compared to soft tissues. The risks related to transmission of high temperatures[52,53] from the skull to the scalp and adjacent brain tissue and the fear of losing the focal spot seemed insurmountable and resulted in invasive procedures, where removal of skull portions was required to clear the sonication pathway. However, the presence of bone and its thickness were not the sole issue. The impedance mismatch between bone and brain tissue additionally distorted the ultrasound beam and shifted its focus; Hynynen and Jolesz[54] were the first to solve this issue, in 1998, combining a multidimensional array with phase correction.[55]

Modern FUS systems have their foundation in these studies further improved by active water cooling, acoustic aberration correction algorithm, and CT data regarding skull thickness/density coregistered between CT and MR images. The treatment protocol is usually divided into 2 different stages: (1) a first stage in which a reversible lesion is created, reaching temperatures in the 45 to 50 °C range and (2) a second and final stage in which

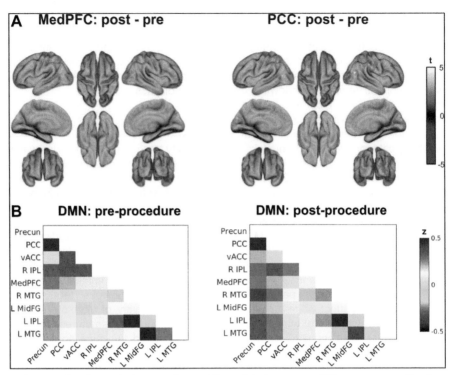

Fig. 1. DMN changes after focused ultrasound central lateral thalamotomy. Difference maps of brain connectivity between preprocedure and 3 months postprocedure of 2 nodes, medial prefrontal cortex and posterior cingulate cortex, to the rest of the brain (post minus pre; *A, B*). DMN, default mode network; L MidFG, left middle frontal gyrus; MedPFC, medial prefrontal cortex; PCC, posterior cingulate cortex; Precun, precuneus; R and L IPL, right and left inferior parietal lobule; R and L MTG, right and left medial temporal gyrus; vACC, ventral anterior cingulate cortex. (*From*: Focused Ultrasound Central Lateral Thalamotomy for the Treatment of Refractory Neuropathic Pain: Phase I Trial, Abdul-Kareem Ahmed, Jiachen Zhuo, Rao P. Gullapalli, and colleagues 2024 Apr 1;94(4):690 to 699. https://doi.org/10.1227/neu.0000000000002752).

a permanent lesion is achieved with temperatures in the 52 to 60 °C range. Peak temperature, duration of events, number of sonication, and amount of applied energy are just a few of the different key points in FUS protocols. In MRgFUS, such as the ExAblate 4000 system (Insightec Inc) which was first approved in 2016 for the treatment of essential tremor,[56] the ability to use MR thermometry not only precisely localizes the anatomic location of the lesion but also allows for supervision of thermal coagulative damage created in real time.[55]

INCISIONLESS THALAMOTOMY THERMOABLATION

Several published studies focus on the use of MRgFUS, targeting various areas of the thalamus specifically for chronic neuropathic pain.

Jeanmonod and colleagues[57] published a nonrandomized prospective observational study, performed in Switzerland approved by the ethics committee of the Zurich University and sponsored by Insightec Ltd. In this pilot study, they included 12 patients, of which 9 were from a previous publication.[58] with 11 successful procedures; one patient was excluded from the analysis as a thermal spot of only 42 °C was obtained in the CL nucleus, not resulting in a thermal ablation lesion. Gallay and colleagues[36] from the same group published a nonrandomized retrospective cross-sectional analysis of all consecutive patients performed between 2011 and 2022, including the 11 from the 2012 observational study. They included 112 CL thalamic targets in 63 interventions with 55 patients, with a mean age at treatment of 62 year (38–80 year). In 7 cases, the contralateral CL thalamic nucleus was the only treated target, while in 48 cases, bilateral CL thalamic nuclei were sonicated. Repeat interventions were required in 8 patients, of which 5 bilaterally and 3 unilaterally. The baseline mean duration of pain was 14 years (3–47 years). Chronic neuropathic pain was due to spinal cord injury (14 subjects), postdiscectomy radiculopathy (6 subjects), thalamic infarction (5 subjects), neuropathy (5 subjects), cortical and basal ganglia infarctions (3 subjects), brainstem injury (3 subjects), plexus avulsion (3 subjects), amputation (2 subjects), postherpetic neuralgia (2 subjects), and chronic cluster headache (1 subject); they also included patients with classical and idiopathic TN (8 subjects) and secondary TN (11 subjects). The mean follow-up duration was 55 months with a range of 3 to 132 months. The authors' assessments were focused on safety and pain relief, the latter via visual analogue scale (VAS) scores and comparison between drug intake at baseline and follow-up. There was one reported serious neurologic event (upper lip numbness and hypoalgesia), during a repeat treatment in a patient who was previously treated with radiofrequency ablation. More than half of the surgeries were painful for a few seconds (56%). The average of VAS scores, respectively, for continuous pain and pain attacks, decreased from 54 ± 16 and 76 ± 16 at baseline to 32 ± 25 and 39 ± 35 at 1 year follow-up, respectively. Opiates drug intake decreased from 32% at baseline to 16% at 1 year follow-up. The authors also showed significant improvement in the quality-of-life World Health Organization Quality-of-Life Scale (WHO-QOL-BREF) questionnaire, Hospital Anxiety and Depression Scale (HADS) scores, and montreal cognitive assessment (MoCA) scores.

Gallay and colleagues[59] also published a retrospective observational study with 180 consecutive MRgFUS treatments and a subgroup of 46 procedures performed to treat CNP. The primary objective of this study was to investigate the safety and accuracy of MRgFUS; pain relief data were also collected but was not part of the analysis. The authors performed pallidothalamic tractotomy ($n = 105$), cerebellothalamic tractotomy ($n = 50$), CL thalamic nucleus ($n = 84$), CM thalamotomy ($n = 12$), and pallidotomy ($n = 2$). There were 4 procedure-related side-effects; benign subcutaneous swelling of the face (2 subjects), right-sided frontal headache (1 subject), and temporal unilateral blindness after supraorbital anesthesia (1 subject). There were 5 non-neurological side-effects (1 lung embolism, 1 cardiac decompensation, 1 bladder infection, 1 patient developed hiccups, and 1 patient had a fall at home 1 week after the procedure). Changes in cognitive status were evaluated through mini–mental state examination (MMSE) and MoCA scores, showing a significant improvement between immediate post-treatment and 1 year follow-up (29.0 ± 1.2 vs 29.4 ± 1.3 and 27.1 ± 2.7 vs 28.0 ± 2.8, respectively). As reported in their previous work,[57] target reconstructions were highly accurate and precise with a mean 3D accuracy of 0.73 ± 0.39 mm.

The prospective, nonrandomized, single-arm, investigator-initiated phase I trial, by Ahmed and colleagues[60] included 10 consecutive patients with 9 successful treatments targeting the CL thalamic nucleus; one patient could not tolerate the procedure because of frame-related pain and prematurely terminated the treatment. CNP was due to radiculopathy (5 subjects), brachial plexus injury (2 subjects), amputation (1 subject), and spinal cord injury (1 subject). The mean age at the time of intervention was 50.9 years (27–69 years). The authors reported no serious adverse events and 12 mild-to-moderate adverse events (headache, pin site tenderness, nausea, blurred vision). Pain relief was assessed at 1 year follow-up using the brief pain inventory (7.6 vs 3.8), the pain disability index (43.0 vs 25.8), and the numeric rating scale (7.2 vs 4.0; **Fig. 2**). In addition, they also assessed functional connectivity analysis pretreatment and posttreatment which showed increased functional connectivity within the DMN.

TECHNICAL ASPECTS AND CHALLENGES

The posterior aspect of the CL nucleus can be consistently identified with advanced imaging. In Ahmed and colleagues' study,[60] planned stereotactic target locations were located 6 to 8 mm cranial to the anterior–posterior commissure plane, 1 mm posterior to 2 mm anterior to the posterior commissure, and 5 to 7 mm lateral to the thalamoventricular border.[57] This target and the nucleus based on Morel's atlas were laid onto 1 mm thick 3 dimensional fast gray matter inversion recovery images. Sagittal and axial images acquired on the day of the procedure were coregistered with prior imaging studies and transducer coordinates (**Fig. 3**).

In the trial,[60] there was no minimum threshold for skull density ratio, and the intent was bilateral treatment. One patient could not tolerate the treatment. Also due to discomfort, another patient only tolerated unilateral treatment. As has been noted in treatment of tremors and Parkinson's, a greater short-duration response (SDR) correlated with lower energy needed for treatment. In this patient population, which is sensitive to discomfort, tolerance for the procedure, which included sitting still on an MR table for 1 to 3 hours, is lower than has been experienced in treating patients for movement disorders.

FUTURE STUDIES

There are currently 5 ongoing studies, studying MRgFUS targets in the thalamus, for the treatment of CNP, not limited to TN: NCT01699477 from the University Children's Hospital of Zurich (nonrandomized, open-label with 30 patients, targeting

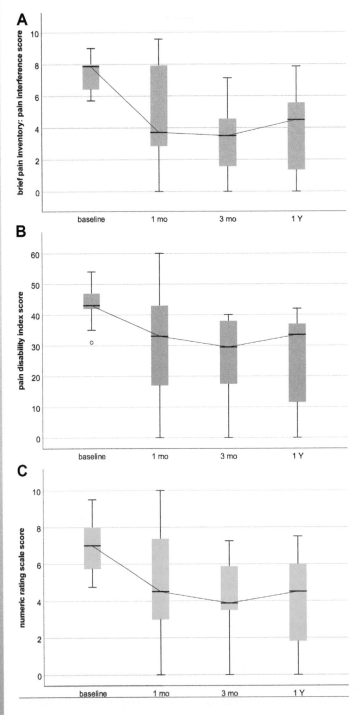

Fig. 2. Pain scores after focused ultrasound central lateral thalamotomy at a 1 year follow-up for 8 patients: brief pain inventory (*A*), pain disability index (*B*), and numeric rating scale (*C*). (*From*: Focused Ultrasound Central Latheral Thalamotomy for the Treatment of Refractory Neuropathic Pain: Phase I Trial, Abdul-Kareem Ahmed, Jiachen Zhuo, Rao P. Gullapalli, and colleagues 2024 Apr 1;94(4):690 to 699. https://doi.org/10.1227/neu.0000000000002752).

the thalamus, subthalamus, and pallidum); NCT04283643 from the University of Virginia (UVA; randomized, parallel-assignment with 149 patients); NCT04485208 from the Neurologic Associates of West Los Angeles (single-group, open-label, 40 patients, targeting the VPM and VPL); NCT04649554 from InSightec Ltd (single-group, open-label, 30 patients); and NCT03100474 (prospective global registry, 500 patients with targets within the thalamus and pallidum).

To summarize the current evidence on MRgFUS, thalamotomy demonstrates that first of all bilateral treatments are generally safe,

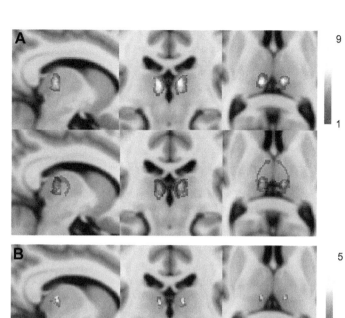

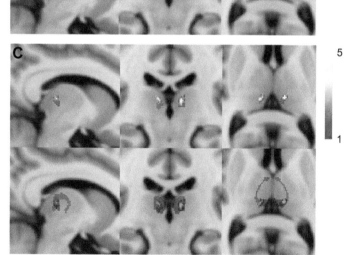

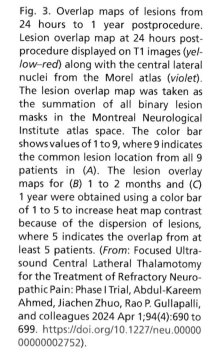

Fig. 3. Overlap maps of lesions from 24 hours to 1 year postprocedure. Lesion overlap map at 24 hours postprocedure displayed on T1 images (*yellow–red*) along with the central lateral nuclei from the Morel atlas (*violet*). The lesion overlap map was taken as the summation of all binary lesion masks in the Montreal Neurological Institute atlas space. The color bar shows values of 1 to 9, where 9 indicates the common lesion location from all 9 patients in (*A*). The lesion overlay maps for (*B*) 1 to 2 months and (*C*) 1 year were obtained using a color bar of 1 to 5 to increase heat map contrast because of the dispersion of lesions, where 5 indicates the overlap from at least 5 patients. (*From*: Focused Ultrasound Central Lathceral Thalamotomy for the Treatment of Refractory Neuropathic Pain: Phase I Trial, Abdul-Kareem Ahmed, Jiachen Zhuo, Rao P. Gullapalli, and colleagues 2024 Apr 1;94(4):690 to 699. https://doi.org/10.1227/neu.0000000000002752).

with mild adverse events and rare permanent somatosensory deficits, especially when targeting the CL thalamic nucleus. When compared with other available treatment options that may lack long-term efficacy, thalamic thermal ablation allows for a more sustained control of pain symptoms with very good results against intermittent pain and allodynia and future efforts should not be limited to this anatomic region. Finally, FUS virtually eliminates the risk of infection.[35,57,61]

MRgFUS may also be more likely to preserve cognitive function as compared to other more invasive interventions[62,63] as shown in the treatment of medically refractory essential tremor. This may be in part related to the ability of FUS to produce smaller and well-focused lesions, leading to overall improvement of patients' wellness.

Although the promising preliminary trends, the vast majority of the data come from retrospective or prospective, nonrandomized, series without controls and with significant heterogeneity between and within subjects regarding the origin of pain.[61]

Thalamotomy for Trigeminal Neuralgia

TN is defined as orofacial pain confined to one or more divisions of the trigeminal nerve, most frequently affecting one side of the face. Its classification was recently revised, identifying three etiologic categories: classical TN, caused by vascular compression of the nerve, secondary TN, caused by major neurologic disease and idiopathic TN, occurring without apparent cause. Current treatment recommendations suggest that microvascular decompression (MVD) may have a weakly better profile when compared to neuroablative treatments in patients with MR-proven nerve compression. Interestingly, no more than a low level of evidence has been shown when considering any lesional intervention (gamma knife, radiofrequency, rhizotomy, and so on) in patients with idiopathic TN.[64]

Gallay and colleagues[65] published a retrospective single-center, case series of 8 consecutive patients with chronic therapy-resistant TN. Using the same technique described in prior publications,[57,59] the bilateral CL thalamic nuclei were the anatomic targets in 6 patients, one patient also received complementation unilateral CL thalamic nucleus, and one additional patient who had previously been treated with bilateral CL thalamic nuclei radiofrequency ablation received unilateral CL thalamic nucleus and CM lesions. The primary outcome was mean pain relief at 3 months (51%), 12 months (71%) and longest follow-up (78%, 4 years mean follow-up length).

The same authors also included patients with TN in a more recent publication, dated 2023[36] where they had a total of 63 patients treated with central lateral thalamic (CLT) including 19 patients with TN. The subgroup analysis showed similar satisfactory results where patients with classical and idiopathic TN ($n = 8$) had a mean pain relief of 76% $\pm$ 19%, while in the subgroup with secondary TN ($n = 11$), the mean pain relief was 31% $\pm$ 42%.

There are currently 3 ongoing studies, exploring MRgFUS targets in the thalamus, for the treatment of TN-related chronic neuropathic pain: NCT04579692 from the University of Maryland, Baltimore (single-group, open-label with 10 patients, targeting the CLT); NCT05122403 from the Chinese PLA General Hospital (case–control with sham, prospective, 12 patients, targeting the CLT); and NCT03309813 from InSightec Ltd (randomized, with sham and potential cross-over after 3 months study visit, 10 patients). Future studies with larger cohorts are needed to demonstrate whether MRgFUS could replace MVD, as a first-line treatment choice in patients with therapy-resistant TN.

Beyond the Thalamus

First described by Foltz and White, surgical cingulotomy was one of the earliest available treatments for refractory pain.[66] A decade later, the stereotactic surgical variation of the technique was introduced by Hurt and Ballantine[67] with modest results. Using the lesson learned from 60s surgeries, Boccard and colleagues[68] and then Levi and colleagues [69] explored the role of dACC deep brain stimulation (DBS), respectively, in CNP and refractory thalamic pain syndrome with satisfactory efficacy metrics.[70]

Emotional salience, learning, reward processing, decision, and empathy as well as the affective aspect of pain are only a few of the higher functions processed by the frontal cingulus.[71–77]

Interestingly, regardless of the specific technique, the mechanism that allows cingulotomy to achieve pain relief is through the management of several neuronal modulation changes, with a strong footprint on the affective, "distress," component of pain.[78] Feng and colleagues[79] successfully targeted the ACC of 54 mice models increasing the mechanical pain withdrawal threshold both in short- and long-term experiments. Shortly after, Wang and colleagues[80] used low-intensity FUS to safely stimulate the ACC, alleviating chronic neuropathic pain-induced allodynia. Strohman and colleagues[81] reported the first series of healthy volunteers to receive low-intensity FUS to the dACC obtained a reduced pain rating when compared to sham.

The mesencephalon is among the other potential stereotactic targets. Between the 1950s and the 1990s, there are a few case series where mesencephalotomy has been used to treat cancer and nonmalignant pain[82–84]; however, this practice has become exceedingly rare in the past couple decades.[85,86] The current most common targets advocate for concurrent interruption of both the lateral and medial pain pathways, transecting the spinothalamic and trigeminothalamic bundles. To the best of our knowledge, the UVA plans to enroll 6 patients with opioid-resistant pain associated with head and neck cancer, with the intent of using FUS to lesion the contralateral mesencephalon and the objective of pain palliation. NCT03894553 is the only ongoing study using MRgFUS in combination with mesencephalotomy and it is designed as a prospective pilot, open-label clinical trial with single-arm treatment.

Thus, FUS targeting the dACC or the mesencephalon may yield helpful anatomic and functional information and future research endeavors may unveil additional anatomic targets.

SUMMARY

Even at its early stages, MRgFUS represents a promising alternative for patients who have failed medical management and other treatment options. The very safe complication profile with low risk of motor and sensory complications and so far anecdotical permanent neurologic deficits make FUS a powerful tool to treat patients otherwise hopeless. Neuromodulation may be the most influential factor driving outcomes and studies devised to detect neuroplasticity will be critical to guide therapies. Future studies should focus on investigating other potential targets, such as the cingulate gyrus or the mesencephalon, as well as integrating control populations in trials.

CLINICS CARE POINTS

- Patients with chronic neuropathic pain have often reached a point where the pain networks will no longer provide a protection mechanism, letting pain become a disease of its own and ultimately culminating in the alteration of the biochemistry of pain transduction.

- The thalamus plays a central role within the complex connections of the pain network, harboring several functional pathways of the pain neuromatrix. Selective targeting of specific thalamic nuclei could restore normal thalamocortical dynamics, affecting the multiple interactions with motor, cognitive, and alerting aspects of pain simultaneously preserving functions supported by other structures.

- MR-guided FUS bilateral treatments are generally safe, with mild adverse events, more sustained control of pain symptoms and rare permanent somatosensory deficits, especially when targeting the central lateral thalamic nucleus.

- MR-guided FUS represents a very safe, promising alternative for patients who have failed medical management and other treatment options. Neuromodulation may be the most influential factor driving outcomes and future studies should focus on investigating the role of neuroplasticity in chronic neuropathic pain.

DISCLOSURE

D. Gandhi reports grants from Microvention, the Focused Ultrasound Foundation, United States, the NIH, United States, and University of Calgary, Canada/Nano Therapeutics. All other authors declared no potential conflicts of interest with respect to the research, authorship, and/or publication of this article.

REFERENCES

1. Terminology | International Association for the Study of Pain. International Association for the Study of Pain (IASP). Available at: https://www.iasp-pain.org/resources/terminology/. [Accessed 27 January 2024].
2. Treede RD, Jensen TS, Campbell JN, et al. Neuropathic pain: redefinition and a grading system for clinical and research purposes. Neurology 2008; 70(18):1630–5.
3. Torrance N, Smith BH, Bennett MI, et al. The epidemiology of chronic pain of predominantly neuropathic origin. Results from a general population survey. J Pain 2006;7(4):281–9.
4. A classification of chronic pain for ICD-11 - PubMed. Available at: https://pubmed.ncbi.nlm.nih.gov/25844555/. [Accessed 27 January 2024].
5. Baek H, Lockwood D, Mason EJ, et al. Clinical intervention using focused ultrasound (FUS) stimulation of the brain in diverse neurological disorders. Front Neurol 2022;13:880814. https://doi.org/10.3389/fneur.2022.880814.
6. Peyron R. [Functional imaging of pain]. Biol Aujourd'hui 2014;208(1):5–12.
7. Tan T, Barry P, Reken S, et al, Guideline Development Group. Pharmacological management of neuropathic pain in non-specialist settings: summary of NICE guidance. BMJ 2010;340:c1079. https://doi.org/10.1136/bmj.c1079.
8. Soldati E. National italian register of implantable systems for spinal cord stimulation (SCS): Analysis of preliminary data. Neuromodulation 2002;5(1):7–15.
9. Cameron T. Safety and efficacy of spinal cord stimulation for the treatment of chronic pain: a 20-year literature review. J Neurosurg 2004;100(3 Suppl Spine):254–67.
10. Franzini A, Ninatti G, Rossini Z, et al. Gamma knife central lateral thalamotomy for chronic neuropathic pain: a single-center, retrospective study. Neurosurgery 2023;92(2):363–9.
11. Franzini A, Attuati L, Zaed I, et al. Gamma Knife central lateral thalamotomy for the treatment of neuropathic pain. J Neurosurg 2020;135(1):228–36.
12. Franzini A, Clerici E, Navarria P, et al. Gamma Knife radiosurgery for the treatment of cluster headache: a systematic review. Neurosurg Rev 2022;45(3): 1923–31.

13. Coffey RJ. Deep brain stimulation for chronic pain: results of two multicenter trials and a structured review. Pain Med 2001;2(3):183–92.

14. Ab Aziz CB, Ahmad AH. The role of the thalamus in modulating pain. Malays J Med Sci 2006;13(2):11–8.

15. Jones AK, Brown WD, Friston KJ, et al. Cortical and subcortical localization of response to pain in man using positron emission tomography. Proc Biol Sci 1991;244(1309):39–44.

16. Yue Y, Collaku A. Correlation of pain reduction with fMRI BOLD Response in osteoarthritis patients treated with paracetamol: randomized, double-blind, crossover clinical efficacy study. Pain Med 2018;19(2):355–67.

17. Rogachov A, Cheng JC, Erpelding N, et al. Regional brain signal variability: a novel indicator of pain sensitivity and coping. Pain 2016;157(11):2483–92.

18. Vamvakas A, Lawn T, Veronese M, et al. Neurotransmitter receptor densities are associated with changes in regional Cerebral blood flow during clinical ongoing pain. Hum Brain Mapp 2022;43(17):5235–49.

19. Melzack R. Pain–an overview. Acta Anaesthesiol Scand 1999;43(9):880–4.

20. Wiech K, Seymour B, Kalisch R, et al. Modulation of pain processing in hyperalgesia by cognitive demand. Neuroimage 2005;27(1):59–69.

21. Omori S, Isose S, Otsuru N, et al. Somatotopic representation of pain in the primary somatosensory cortex (S1) in humans. Clin Neurophysiol 2013;124(7):1422–30.

22. Ferretti A, Del Gratta C, Babiloni C, et al. Functional topography of the secondary somatosensory cortex for nonpainful and painful stimulation of median and tibial nerve: an fMRI study. Neuroimage 2004;23(3):1217–25.

23. Ploner M, Schmitz F, Freund HJ, et al. Parallel activation of primary and secondary somatosensory cortices in human pain processing. J Neurophysiol 1999;81(6):3100–4.

24. Apkarian AV, Bushnell MC, Treede RD, et al. Human brain mechanisms of pain perception and regulation in health and disease. Eur J Pain 2005;9(4):463–84.

25. Vogt BA, Berger GR, Derbyshire SWG. Structural and functional dichotomy of human midcingulate cortex. Eur J Neurosci 2003;18(11):3134–44.

26. Russo JF, Sheth SA. Deep brain stimulation of the dorsal anterior cingulate cortex for the treatment of chronic neuropathic pain. Neurosurg Focus 2015;38(6):E11. https://doi.org/10.3171/2015.3.FOCUS1543.

27. Mazzola L, Isnard J, Peyron R, et al. Stimulation of the human cortex and the experience of pain: Wilder Penfield's observations revisited. Brain 2012;135(Pt 2):631–40.

28. Perrotta A, Chiacchiaretta P, Anastasio MG, et al. Temporal summation of the nociceptive withdrawal reflex involves deactivation of posterior cingulate cortex. Eur J Pain 2017;21(2):289–301.

29. Nüssel M, Zhao Y, Knorr C, et al. Deep brain stimulation, stereotactic radiosurgery and high-intensity focused ultrasound targeting the limbic pain matrix: A comprehensive review. Pain Ther 2022;11(2):459–76.

30. Georgescu IA, Popa D, Zagrean L. The anatomical and functional heterogeneity of the mediodorsal thalamus. Brain Sci 2020;10(9):624.

31. Mitchell A, Chakraborty S. What does the mediodorsal thalamus do? Front Syst Neurosci 2013;7. Available at: https://www.frontiersin.org/articles/10.3389/fnsys.2013.00037. [Accessed 28 February 2024].

32. Cappe C, Rouiller EM, Barone P. Cortical and thalamic pathways for multisensory and sensorimotor interplay. In: Murray MM, Wallace MT, editors. The neural bases of multisensory processes. frontiers in neuroscience. CRC Press/Taylor & Francis; 2012. Available at: http://www.ncbi.nlm.nih.gov/books/NBK92866/. [Accessed 28 February 2024].

33. Richardson DE. Thalamotomy for intractable pain. Confin Neurol 1967;29(2):139–45.

34. Jeanmonod D, Morel A. The central lateral thalamotomy for neuropathic pain. In: Lozano AM, Gildenberg PL, Tasker RR, editors. Textbook of stereotactic and functional neurosurgery. Springer; 2009. p. 2081–96. https://doi.org/10.1007/978-3-540-69960-6_123.

35. Jeanmonod D, Magnin M, Morel A, et al. Surgical control of the human thalamocortical dysrhythmia:: I. Central lateral thalamotomy in neurogenic pain. Thalamus Relat Syst 2001;1(1):71–9.

36. Gallay MN, Magara AE, Moser D, et al. Magnetic resonance-guided focused ultrasound central lateral thalamotomy against chronic and therapy-resistant neuropathic pain: retrospective long-term follow-up analysis of 63 interventions. J Neurosurg 2023;139(3):615–24.

37. Sarnthein J, Stern J, Aufenberg C, et al. Increased EEG power and slowed dominant frequency in patients with neurogenic pain. Brain 2006;129(Pt 1):55–64.

38. Llinás RR, Ribary U, Jeanmonod D, et al. Thalamocortical dysrhythmia: A neurological and neuropsychiatric syndrome characterized by magnetoencephalography. Proc Natl Acad Sci USA 1999;96(26):15222–7.

39. Bastuji H, Frot M, Mazza S, et al. Thalamic responses to nociceptive-specific input in humans: functional dichotomies and thalamocortical connectivity. Cereb Cortex 2016;26(6):2663–76.

40. Albe-Fessard D, Berkley KJ, Kruger L, et al. Diencephalic mechanisms of pain sensation. Brain Res 1985;356(3):217–96.

41. Tagliazucchi E, Balenzuela P, Fraiman D, et al. Brain resting state is disrupted in chronic back pain patients. Neurosci Lett 2010;485(1):26–31.

42. Morton DL, Sandhu JS, Jones AK. Brain imaging of pain: state of the art. J Pain Res 2016;9:613–24.
43. Baliki MN, Mansour AR, Baria AT, et al. Functional reorganization of the default mode network across chronic pain conditions. PLoS One 2014;9(9): e106133. https://doi.org/10.1371/journal.pone. 0106133.
44. Fry FJ. Ultrasonic visualization of human brain structure. Invest Radiol 1970;5(2):117–21.
45. Fry WJ, Barnard JW, Fry FJ, et al. Ultrasonically produced localized selective lesions in the central nervous system. Am J Phys Med 1955;34(3): 413–23.
46. Fry WJ, Mosberg WH, Barnard JW, et al. Production of focal destructive lesions in the central nervous system with ultrasound. J Neurosurg 1954;11(5): 471–8.
47. Lele PP. Production of deep focal lesions by focused ultrasound–current status. Ultrasonics 1967;5: 105–12.
48. Lynn JG, Zwemer RL, Chick AJ, et al. A new method for the generation and use of focused ultrasound in experimental biology. J Gen Physiol 1942;26(2): 179–93.
49. D'Andrea A, Conte M, Scarafile R, et al. Transcranial doppler ultrasound: physical principles and principal applications in neurocritical care unit. J Cardiovasc Echogr 2016;26(2):28–41.
50. Marinoni M, Ginanneschi A, Forleo P, et al. Technical limits in transcranial Doppler recording: inadequate acoustic windows. Ultrasound Med Biol 1997; 23(8):1275–7.
51. Aaslid R, Markwalder TM, Nornes H. Noninvasive transcranial Doppler ultrasound recording of flow velocity in basal cerebral arteries. J Neurosurg 1982;57(6):769–74.
52. Guthkelch AN, Carter LP, Cassady JR, et al. Treatment of malignant brain tumors with focused ultrasound hyperthermia and radiation: results of a phase I trial. J Neuro Oncol 1991;10(3):271–84.
53. McDannold N, Clement GT, Black P, et al. Transcranial magnetic resonance imaging- guided focused ultrasound surgery of brain tumors: initial findings in 3 patients. Neurosurgery 2010;66(2):323–32 [discussion: 332].
54. Hynynen K, Jolesz FA. Demonstration of potential noninvasive ultrasound brain therapy through an intact skull. Ultrasound Med Biol 1998;24(2):275–83.
55. Harary M, Segar DJ, Huang KT, et al. Focused ultrasound in neurosurgery: a historical perspective. Neurosurg Focus 2018;44(2):E2.
56. Elias WJ, Huss D, Voss T, et al. A pilot study of focused ultrasound thalamotomy for essential tremor. N Engl J Med 2013;369(7):640–8.
57. Jeanmonod D, Werner B, Morel A, et al. Transcranial magnetic resonance imaging-guided focused ultrasound: noninvasive central lateral thalamotomy for chronic neuropathic pain. Neurosurg Focus 2012;32(1): E1. https://doi.org/10.3171/2011.10.FOCUS11248.
58. Martin E, Jeanmonod D, Morel A, et al. High-intensity focused ultrasound for noninvasive functional neurosurgery. Ann Neurol 2009;66(6):858–61.
59. Gallay MN, Moser D, Jeanmonod D. Safety and accuracy of incisionless transcranial MR-guided focused ultrasound functional neurosurgery: single-center experience with 253 targets in 180 treatments. J Neurosurg 2018;130(4):1234–43.
60. Ahmed AK, Zhuo J, Gullapalli RP, et al. Focused ultrasound central lateral thalamotomy for the treatment of refractory neuropathic pain: Phase I trial. Neurosurgery 2023. https://doi.org/10.1227/neu. 0000000000002752.
61. Kinfe T. MR-guided high-intensity focused ultrasound for chronic pain: where do we stand? Expert Rev Neurother 2023;23(9):757–61.
62. Saporito G, Sucapane P, Ornello R, et al. Cognitive outcomes after focused ultrasound thalamotomy for tremor: Results from the COGNIFUS (COGNitive in Focused UltraSound) study. Parkinsonism Relat Disorders 2023;106:105230. https://doi.org/10. 1016/j.parkreldis.2022.105230.
63. Pirrotta R, Jeanmonod D, McAleese S, et al. Cognitive functioning, emotional processing, mood, and personality variables before and after stereotactic surgery: a study of 8 cases with chronic neuropathic pain. Neurosurgery 2013;73(1):121–8.
64. Bendtsen L, Zakrzewska JM, Abbott J, et al. European academy of neurology guideline on trigeminal neuralgia. Eur J Neurol 2019;26(6):831–49.
65. Gallay MN, Moser D, Jeanmonod D. MR-guided focused ultrasound central lateral thalamotomy for trigeminal neuralgia. Single center experience. Front Neurol 2020;11:271.
66. Foltz EL, White LE. Pain "relief" by frontal cingulumotomy. J Neurosurg 1962;19:89–100.
67. Hurt RW, Ballantine HT. Stereotactic anterior cingulate lesions for persistent pain: a report on 68 cases. Clin Neurosurg 1974;21:334–51.
68. Boccard SGJ, Pereira EAC, Moir L, et al. Deep brain stimulation of the anterior cingulate cortex: targeting the affective component of chronic pain. Neuroreport 2014;25(2):83–8.
69. Levi V, Cordella R, D'Ammando A, et al. Dorsal anterior cingulate cortex (ACC) deep brain stimulation (DBS): a promising surgical option for the treatment of refractory thalamic pain syndrome (TPS). Acta Neurochir 2019;161(8):1579–88.
70. Spangler WJ, Cosgrove GR, Ballantine HT, et al. Magnetic resonance image-guided stereotactic cingulotomy for intractable psychiatric disease. Neurosurgery 1996;38(6):1071–6 [discussion: 1076-1078].
71. Apkarian AV, Neugebauer V, Koob G, et al. Neural mechanisms of pain and alcohol dependence. Pharmacol Biochem Behav 2013;112:34–41.

72. Bechara A, Damasio AR, Damasio H, et al. Insensitivity to future consequences following damage to human prefrontal cortex. Cognition 1994;50(1–3): 7–15.

73. Cohen MX, Heller AS, Ranganath C. Functional connectivity with anterior cingulate and orbitofrontal cortices during decision-making. Brain Res Cogn Brain Res. 2005;23(1):61–70.

74. Cohen RA, Kaplan RF, Moser DJ, et al. Impairments of attention after cingulotomy. Neurology 1999;53(4): 819–24.

75. Devinsky O, Morrell MJ, Vogt BA. Contributions of anterior cingulate cortex to behaviour. Brain 1995; 118(Pt 1):279–306.

76. Qu C, King T, Okun A, et al. Lesion of the rostral anterior cingulate cortex eliminates the aversiveness of spontaneous neuropathic pain following partial or complete axotomy. Pain 2011;152(7):1641–8.

77. Jahn A, Nee DE, Alexander WH, et al. Distinct regions of anterior cingulate cortex signal prediction and outcome evaluation. Neuroimage 2014;95:80–9.

78. Farrell SM, Green A, Aziz T. The current state of deep brain stimulation for chronic pain and its context in other forms of neuromodulation. Brain Sci 2018;8(8):158.

79. Feng X, Niu L, Long M, et al. Transcranial ultrasound stimulation of the anterior cingulate cortex reduces neuropathic pain in mice. Evid Based Complement Alternat Med 2021;2021:6510383. https://doi.org/10.1155/2021/6510383.

80. Wang B, Chen MX, Chen SC, et al. Low-intensity focused ultrasound alleviates chronic neuropathic pain-induced allodynia by inhibiting neuroplasticity in the anterior cingulate cortex. Neural Plast 2022; 2022. https://doi.org/10.1155/2022/6472475.

81. Strohman A, Payne B, In A, et al. Low-intensity focused ultrasound to the human dorsal anterior cingulate attenuates acute pain perception and autonomic responses. J Neurosci 2024;44: e1011232023.

82. Amano K, Kawamura H, Tanikawa T, et al. Stereotactic mesencephalotomy for pain relief. A plea for stereotactic surgery. Stereotact Funct Neurosurg 1992; 59(1–4):25–32.

83. Frank F, Tognetti F, Gaist G, et al. Stereotaxic rostral mesencephalotomy in treatment of malignant facio-thoracobrachial pain syndromes. A survey of 14 treated patients. J Neurosurg 1982;56(6):807–11.

84. Whisler WW, Voris HC. Mesencephalotomy for intractable pain due to malignant disease. Appl Neurophysiol 1978;41(1–4):52–6.

85. Ivanishvili Z, Pujara S, Honey CM, et al. Stereotactic mesencephalotomy for palliative care pain control: A case report, literature review and plea to rediscover this operation. Br J Neurosurg 2016;30(4): 444–7.

86. Marques RAS, Alencar HS, Bannach MA, et al. Semidirect targeting-based stereotactic mesencephalotomy for the treatment of refractory pain: a case series. J Neurosurg 2022;136(4):1128–38.

MR Imaging–Guided Focused Ultrasound— Clinical Applications in Managing Malignant Gliomas

Huanwen Chen, MD[a], Pavlos Anastasiadis, PhD[b,c],
Graeme F. Woodworth, MD[b,c],*

KEYWORDS

- Glioma • Glioblastoma • Ultrasound • Sonodynamic therapy • Ablation • MR imaging
- Blood-brain barrier • Immunotherapy

KEY POINTS

- MR imaging–guided focused ultrasound (MRgFUS) is an emerging noninvasive technology with great promise for managing malignant gliomas.
- MRgFUS can induce direct tumor cell killing by thermal ablation, histotripsy, or sonodynamic therapy.
- MRgFUS can open the blood-brain barrier to facilitate the delivery of therapeutic agents into the tumor and the release of tumor antigens and genetic materials into the systemic circulation.
- MRgFUS can also modulate the tumor immune microenvironment to augment antitumor immunity.

INTRODUCTION

Malignant gliomas (MGs), including glioblastoma (GBM), are the most aggressive and common forms of primary brain tumors in adults, presenting a significant challenge in neuro-oncology. The global incidence is approximately 3 per 100,000 individuals annually, with a slight male predominance.[1] Despite advances in our understanding and management of these tumors, the prognosis remains dismal, with a median survival of approximately 15 months for GBM patients.[2]

Current standard treatment for MGs involves maximal safe surgical resection followed by concurrent radiotherapy and temozolomide (TMZ) chemotherapy, a regimen that improves survival by 2.5 months.[2] However, while successful surgical removal of MGs improves overall patient survival,

safe total resection is not always feasible. This is particularly true for tumors in deep-seated or eloquent brain regions (eg, brainstem).[3] Furthermore, the nearly universal recurrence of the disease necessitates additional treatments, often involving repeat surgery, re-irradiation, and second-line chemotherapy or experimental therapies.

Recent advances in molecular biology and genomics have paved the way for developing targeted therapies for specific genetic and molecular vulnerabilities in gliomas. Agents targeting the epidermal growth factor receptor (EGFR), which is frequently amplified and mutated in GBM, and the vascular endothelial growth factor pathway, crucial for the tumor's angiogenesis, have been extensively studied; however, clinical trials of targeted agents have so far failed to demonstrate a significant survival benefit, underscoring the challenges posed by

a National Institute of Neurological Disorders and Stroke, National Institutes of Health, 10 Center Drive, Bethesda, MD 20892, USA; b Department of Neurosurgery, University of Maryland School of Medicine, S-12D, 22 South Greene Street, Baltimore, MD 21201, USA; c University of Maryland Marlene and Stewart Greenebaum Comprehensive Cancer Center
* Corresponding author. Department of Neurosurgery, S-12D, 22 South Greene Street, Baltimore, MD 21201.
E-mail address: gwoodworth@som.umaryland.edu

Magn Reson Imaging Clin N Am 32 (2024) 673–679
https://doi.org/10.1016/j.mric.2024.05.006
1064-9689/24/© 2024 Elsevier Inc. All rights are reserved, including those for text and data mining, AI training, and similar technologies.

GBM heterogeneity and the impediments to drug delivery, in particular the blood-brain barrier (BBB).[4,5] Immunotherapy, including checkpoint inhibitors, vaccines, and adoptive cell therapies, also represents a promising new frontier in glioma treatment, although results have been mixed.[6] The heterogeneity of gliomas, inter-tumorally and intra-tumorally, along with the immunosuppressive tumor microenvironment, presents significant obstacles to the effectiveness of these therapies.[6] Thus, developing more effective treatments for MGs remains an area of active research, and there is an increasing focus on overcoming the challenges of drug and therapeutic delivery across the BBB.[6]

MR imaging–guided focused ultrasound (MRgFUS) is an emerging noninvasive technology with great promise for managing MGs. In this review, the authors highlight the potential uses of MRgFUS to induce tumor cell death, modulate the BBB, and facilitate the release of tumor genetic and molecular markers into the peripheral blood circulation for diagnostic use. The authors also discuss the intricate cross talk between FUS applications and the tumor immune microenvironment for MGs.

PRINCIPLES OF FOCUSED ULTRASOUND

Although the origins of FUS for brain applications extend back to the mid-twentieth century, it was not until recently that FUS was combined with MR guidance for treating brain diseases. FUS modalities leverage thermal and mechanical effects to modulate target tissues with minimal effects on surrounding healthy structures. To generate thermal effects, continuous or long bursts of ultrasound at moderately high intensity and high duty cycle are emitted from an array of transducers.[7] At lower temperatures, tissue hyperthermia can increase vascular perfusion, potentially sensitizing tumors to treatments.[8,9] In particular, FUS can induce local hyperthermia below the threshold required for coagulative necrosis and can augment tissue oxygenation and perfusion, thereby sensitizing tissue to radiation therapy.[10–12] Thermal stress occurs at ultrasound intensities larger than 10 W/cm[13] due to friction at the molecular level within tissues as the molecules become out of phase with the propagating pressure wave (eg, viscous heating). By modulating the amplitude, pulse duration, and duty cycle, different levels of heat can be achieved, from mild hyperthermia (<43 °C) to thermal ablation (~60 °C).[14] A clinical trial is currently underway to investigate the radiosensitization effects of FUS-induced hyperthermia (NCT04988750). Temperature changes can be monitored in real time with MR thermometry, providing immediate feedback to track treatment effects.[15]

TUMOR CELL KILLING

One of the main benefits of FUS-induced tumor cell killing is its noninvasive nature, limiting the risks associated with surgery (eg, infection) and shortening recovery times. Furthermore, the ability of MRgFUS to precisely target and ablate tumor tissues without affecting adjacent healthy cells holds the potential for reduced side effects compared to traditional treatments like radiation therapy and chemotherapy. This precision also allows for treating tumors considered inoperable due to their location. Three primary FUS-mediated tumor cell–killing mechanisms exist: thermal ablation, histotripsy, and sonodynamic therapy (SDT).

Thermal Ablation

High-intensity FUS (HIFU) can induce cell death by thermal effects.[16] By concentrating continuous ultrasound waves to a focal point, HIFU can induce thermal ablation of targeted tissues, causing cell death in a precise volume without damaging surrounding structures. The treatment effects of HIFU thermal ablation can be visualized in real time with MR thermometry, and the overall feasibility of MR-guided HIFU was demonstrated in rats[17,18] and pigs,[19] where thermal ablation led to precise destruction of predefined brain areas with minimal perilesion damage or edema. In 2006, Ram and colleagues[20] treated 3 recurrent GBM patients with HIFU thermal ablation and achieved resolution of enhancement in the treated volume of 2 patients. Subsequently, McDannold and colleagues[21] attempted MR-guided HIFU thermal ablation for 3 GBM patients in 2010 using the ExAblate 3000 system; the maximum focal temperature achieved during a 20-second sonication was approximately 51°C, clearly below the threshold for thermal damage in the brain. There was no evidence of tissue, skull, or tumor changes due to the treatment.[22]

Histotripsy

FUS can also be used as a mechanical and nonthermal ablation method that uses short, high-intensity ultrasound pulses, typically in the microsecond range, to generate cavitation microbubble (MB) clouds that fractionate tissue, also termed histotripsy.[23] Histotripsy has been investigated as a treatment modality for brain tumors. Hemispherical transcranial histotripsy transducer arrays (250 and 500 kHz) with 256 elements and a focal distance of 15 cm were designed and tested using *ex vivo* bovine brains.[24] This *ex vivo* model demonstrated that histotripsy could ablate deep structures in the brain. Multiple *in vivo* preclinical studies have shown that histotripsy can reliably create lesions in the brain. In a porcine model, Sukovich and colleagues[25] demonstrated that histotripsy could generate predefined and arbitrarily shaped lesions in pigs, sparing perilesional tissue beyond 200 microns from the histotripsy margin. However, concerns that mechanical tissue disruption induced by histotripsy could induce hemorrhages or edema in the brain have impeded the use of histotripsy for brain indications.[7]

Sonodynamic Therapy

MRgFUS can also be used at low intensity in conjunction with sonosensitizing agents that preferentially accumulate in tumor cells, which, with the collapse of cavitation MBs generated by pulsed FUS, lead to the creation of reactive oxygen species that in turn induces tumor cell death. Compared to thermal ablation and histotripsy, SDT carries an inherently lower risk of causing cavitary lesions and hemorrhagic complications, which may be an advantage for the treatment of intracranial tumors, particularly in deep-seated locations. Various sonosensitizers, including 5-aminolevulinic acid (5-ALA) and fluorescein, have shown promise in preclinical models. Wu and colleagues[26] showed that SDT with MRgFUS and 5-ALA induced apoptosis and suppressed tumor proliferation in a rat glioma model. Yoshida and colleagues[27] reported similar findings using the ExAblate 4000 MRgFUS system. Prada and colleagues[28] also demonstrated the potential promise of SDT with MRgFUS and fluorescein using a rat ectopic MG model. TMZ, the mainstay chemotherapeutic agent for MGs, can also be used as a sonosensitizer using a liposomal drug delivery platform, and Zhou and colleagues[29] demonstrated that TMZ-based SDT may facilitate the induction of immunogenic cell death. Other sonosensitizers, such as sinoporphyrin sodium, hematoporphyrin monomethyl ether, and rose bengal, have also been investigated in preclinical animal models, generally demonstrating promising results.[30] Multiple clinical trials using 5-ALA-based SDT are currently underway (NCT06039709, NCT04845919, NCT04559685, NCT05123534, NCT05370508, NCT05362409), and results are eagerly awaited.

FOCUSED ULTRASOUND–ENABLED BLOOD-BRAIN BARRIER OPENING

The ability of MRgFUS to modulate the BBB in a noninvasive fashion has attracted increased attention for various brain pathologies beyond malignancies, including Alzheimer's disease and amyotrophic lateral sclerosis. Here, the interaction of intravenously circulating MBs with ultrasound waves causes MBs to undergo repetitive rarefaction and expansion in response to the ultrasound, temporarily disrupting the tight junctions of the cerebral endothelium, thereby leading to transient BBB opening. In 2001, Hynynen and colleagues[31] demonstrated in rabbits that MR-guided, low-intensity, pulsed FUS in conjunction with intravenously injected ultrasonographic contrast can induce transient opening of the BBB without damage to neuronal tissue. Notably, BBB opening was transient, as evidenced by a lack of contrast enhancement 1 day after the initial FUS procedure.[31] Subsequent studies further demonstrated the feasibility of MRgFUS-mediated BBB opening, confirming the consistent effectiveness and minimal safety concerns in animal models.[21,22,31] MRgFUS-mediated BBB opening for MGs enables the enhanced delivery of therapeutic agents into the tumor.

Focused Ultrasound–Mediated Drug Delivery

MRgFUS has been used in several studies to modulate the BBB for glioma patients and facilitate the delivery of chemotherapeutic agents. In 2019, Idbaih and colleagues[32] used an implanted pulsed ultrasound system to induce BBB opening and enhance carboplatin penetration in 19 GBM patients; results demonstrated that ultrasound-mediated BBB opening was well tolerated and may improve chemotherapeutic delivery. Mainprize and colleagues[33] also showed that MRgFUS achieved similar results in 5 patients with confirmed or suspected high-grade glioma who underwent sonication with liposomal doxorubicin and TMZ treatments. Additional clinical trials are underway investigating FUS-mediated BBB opening and its effect on chemotherapeutic delivery (NCT 05762419, NCT05630209, NCT05615623). FUS-facilitated BBB opening may also enhance the delivery of other therapeutics, such as viral vectors, gene therapy, and nanotherapeutics,[34–37] pending further research.

Focused Ultrasound–Enabled Liquid Biopsy

Integrating molecular and genetic tumor profiling into clinical practice may enable a more personalized approach to therapy that could lead to improved outcomes.[38,39] In this setting, BBB opening can facilitate liquid biopsy by releasing tumor-derived DNA and other biomarkers into the systemic blood circulation. This can be used as a noninvasive means of profiling MG molecular and genetic signatures. In a mouse model of enhanced green fluorescent protein (eGFP)–transduced GBM, FUS was shown to increase the amount of eGFP messenger RNA in the peripheral circulation, suggesting that FUS-induced BBB opening may be associated with the hematologic release of tumor genetic material.[40] In a separate study using mouse and pig GBM models, Pacia and colleagues[41] showed that MRgFUS opening of the BBB substantially increased the detectability of EGFR variant III and telomerase reverse transcriptase C228 T mutations in the peripheral circulation,[42] which are clinically critical molecular signatures for glioma patients. Clinical trials investigating the utility of BBB opening to facilitate liquid biopsy for GBM patients (NCT05383872) are underway.

FOCUSED ULTRASOUND–MEDIATED IMMUNOMODULATION

Tumor cell death leads to a release of tumor antigens, which primes the immune system to recognize other tumor cells, leading to further tumor cell killing. For MGs, however, multiple barriers exist. The trafficking of tumor antigens or tumor-derived tumor DNA into the systemic circulation is impeded by the BBB.[43] Moreover, the molecular signatures of MGs and their surface antigens are highly heterogeneous and diverse,[44] which could impede efficient antigen spread and continued propagation of the tumor immune microenvironment. Brain tumors may be associated with local and systemic immunosuppression.[45–47] Finally, chemotherapeutic agents, radiation, and corticosteroids used to treat MGs also have inadvertent immunosuppressive effects.[48–50]

Applications of FUS can modulate the tumor immune responses through several mechanisms. First, FUS ablation can lead to various downstream immunomodulatory effects.[16] For one, FUS ablation can trigger the release of tumor antigens previously sequestered within the brain tumor microenvironment, enhance antigen presentation, and stimulate the activation of the adaptive immune response against tumors.[16] Furthermore, FUS can induce a form of immunogenic cell death in tumor cells, characterized by the release of damage-associated molecular patterns (DAMPs); these DAMPs can further stimulate the immune system by enhancing dendritic cell maturation and T-cell activation, promoting a more robust antitumor immune response.[16] FUS ablation has been shown to increase immune cell infiltration and augment T-lymphocyte cytotoxicity in tumors in preclinical models.[51–54] Clinical studies have also demonstrated the proinflammatory and immunogenic effects of FUS ablation in various cancers.[16]

For gliomas, FUS-induced hyperthermia may have unique immunologic implications; in an in vitro model for murine glioma cells, Sheybani and colleagues[55] demonstrated that FUS-induced hyperthermia augmented the release of extracellular vesicles by 46%; furthermore, the vesicles released after FUS-induced hyperthermia led to significant upregulation of interleukin (IL)-12p70 in dendritic cells, consistent with a proinflammatory stimulus. SDT may also modulate the tumor immune microenvironment; using a mouse glioma model, Pellegatta and colleagues[56] showed that fluorescein-mediated SDT leads to the depletion of myeloid-derived suppressor cells, resulting in an overall immunostimulatory effect. Finally, the FUS opening of the BBB can also directly modulate the tumor immune microenvironment, facilitate the infiltration of immune effector cells, and allow tumor antigens to enter the systemic circulation. Kovacs and colleagues[57] suggested that FUS in a rodent model induces the release of DAMPs, stimulating a local sterile inflammatory response that may also modulate the tumor immune microenvironment. In another study, Sheybani and colleagues[41] suggested that BBB opening with MRgFUS increases the recruitment of dendritic cells, which could augment the activation of adaptive tumor immunity.

Using a patient-derived xenograft mouse model of MG, Brighi and colleagues[58] showed that BBB opening with FUS could facilitate tumor penetration of antibodies, particularly in tumor regions that were not contrast-enhancing. In another mouse glioma model, Sabbagh and colleagues[59] showed that BBB opening with pulsed ultrasound might augment the therapeutic efficacy of anti-programmed cell death protein 1 monoclonal antibodies and chimeric antigen receptor T cells. Finally, Chen and colleagues[60] also demonstrated in a rat glioma model that BBB opening using FUS can enhance the effects of intra-tumoral IL-12 delivery and augment the subsequent recruitment of immune effector cells. Clinical trials are underway to investigate whether FUS-mediated BBB opening may enhance the therapeutic efficacy of bevacizumab (NCT06329570) and pembrolizumab (NCT05879120).

SUMMARY

FUS is a rapidly evolving, promising technology for treating brain malignancies noninvasively. Various potential applications in managing MGs are being studied, including thermal ablation, histotripsy, SDT, BBB opening, and immune modulation. FUS clinical trials thus far have primarily focused on feasibility and safety. Notably, the ability of

FUS to modulate the tumor immune microenvironment in the brain makes it ideal for combination therapies with immunotherapeutic agents, such as cellular therapy, checkpoint inhibitors, and cancer vaccines. By enhancing tumor antigen release, immune cell infiltration, and drug entry, FUS can overcome the immunosuppressive barriers that convert the tumor immune microenvironment and limit the efficacy of immunotherapy in brain tumors. Early preclinical and clinical studies have begun to explore these combinations, showing promising results in improving overall treatment efficacy.

CLINICS CARE POINTS

- MRgFUS has shown great promise in preclinical models and early clinical trials.
- Multiple clinical trials for MRgFUS applications, specifically SDT and BBB opening, are underway.
- Future studies are needed to explore further how MRgFUS applications can be used to optimize existing or experimental therapeutics.

DISCLOSURE

The authors have no relevant disclosures.

FUNDING

G.F. Woodworth: R01NS107813; R01CA269995. P. Anastasiadis: Seed Funds from the Department of Neurosurgery, University of Maryland School of Medicine, and the American Cancer Society's Institutional Research Grant IRG-18-160-16.

REFERENCES

1. Ostrom QT, Gittleman H, Liao P, et al. CBTRUS statistical report: primary brain and central nervous system tumors diagnosed in the United States in 2007-2011. Neuro Oncol 2014;16(Suppl 4):iv1–63.
2. Stupp R, Mason WP, van den Bent MJ, et al. Radiotherapy plus concomitant and adjuvant temozolomide for glioblastoma. N Engl J Med 2005;352:987–96.
3. Karschnia P, Vogelbaum MA, van den Bent M, et al. Evidence-based recommendations on categories for extent of resection in diffuse glioma. Eur J Cancer 2021;149:23–33.
4. Chen H, Kuhn J, Lamborn KR, et al. Phase I/II study of sorafenib in combination with erlotinib for recurrent glioblastoma as part of a 3-arm sequential accrual clinical trial: NABTC 05-02. Neurooncol Adv 2020;2:vdaa124.
5. Begagić E, Pugonja R, Bečulić H, et al. Molecular Targeted Therapies in Glioblastoma Multiforme: A Systematic Overview of Global Trends and Findings. Brain Sci 2023;13(11):1602.
6. Lim M, Xia Y, Bettegowda C, et al. Current state of immunotherapy for glioblastoma. Nat Rev Clin Oncol 2018;15:422–42.
7. Xu Z, Hall TL, Vlaisavljevich E, et al. Histotripsy: the first noninvasive, non-ionizing, non-thermal ablation technique based on ultrasound. Int J Hyperthermia 2021;38:561–75.
8. Tretbar SH, Fournelle M, Speicher D, et al. A Novel Matrix-Array-Based MR-Conditional Ultrasound System for Local Hyperthermia of Small Animals. IEEE Trans Biomed Eng 2022;69:758–70.
9. Chan H, Chang H-Y, Lin W-L, et al. Large-Volume Focused-Ultrasound Mild Hyperthermia for Improving Blood-Brain Tumor Barrier Permeability Application. Pharmaceutics 2022;14(10):2012.
10. Hu S, Zhang X, Unger M, et al. Focused Ultrasound-Induced Cavitation Sensitizes Cancer Cells to Radiation Therapy and Hyperthermia. Cells 2020;9(12):2595.
11. Zhu L, Altman MB, Laszlo A, et al. Ultrasound Hyperthermia Technology for Radiosensitization. Ultrasound Med Biol 2019;45:1025–43.
12. Schneider CS, Woodworth GF, Vujaskovic Z, et al. Radiosensitization of high-grade gliomas through induced hyperthermia: Review of clinical experience and the potential role of MR-guided focused ultrasound. Radiother Oncol 2020;142:43–51.
13. ter Haar G. Therapeutic applications of ultrasound. Prog Biophys Mol Biol 2007;93:111–29.
14. Kim C, Lim M, Woodworth GF, et al. The roles of thermal and mechanical stress in focused ultrasound-mediated immunomodulation and immunotherapy for central nervous system tumors. J Neuro Oncol 2022;157:221–36.
15. Odéen H, Parker DL. Magnetic resonance thermometry and its biological applications - Physical principles and practical considerations. Prog Nucl Magn Reson Spectrosc 2019;110:34–61.
16. van den Bijgaart RJE, Eikelenboom DC, Hoogenboom M, et al. Thermal and mechanical high-intensity focused ultrasound: perspectives on tumor ablation, immune effects and combination strategies. Cancer Immunol Immunother 2017;66:247–58.
17. Dervishi E, Larrat B, Pernot M, et al. Transcranial high intensity focused ultrasound therapy guided by 7 TESLA MRI in a rat brain tumour model: a feasibility study. Int J Hyperthermia 2013;29:598–608.
18. Hijnen NM, Heijman E, Köhler MO, et al. Tumour hyperthermia and ablation in rats using a clinical

MR-HIFU system equipped with a dedicated small animal set-up. Int J Hyperthermia 2012;28:141–55.

19. Cohen ZR, Zaubermann J, Harnof S, et al. Magnetic resonance imaging-guided focused ultrasound for thermal ablation in the brain: a feasibility study in a swine model. Neurosurgery 2007;60:593–600. ; discussion 600.

20. Ram Z, Cohen ZR, Harnof S, et al. Magnetic resonance imaging-guided, high-intensity focused ultrasound for brain tumor therapy. Neurosurgery 2006;59(5):949–55.

21. McDannold N, Vykhodtseva N, Jolesz FA, et al. MRI investigation of the threshold for thermally induced blood-brain barrier disruption and brain tissue damage in the rabbit brain. Magn Reson Med 2004;51:913–23.

22. McDannold N, Clement GT, Black P, et al. Transcranial magnetic resonance imaging- guided focused ultrasound surgery of brain tumors: initial findings in 3 patients. Neurosurgery 2010;66:323–32. discussion 332.

23. Roberts WW. Development and translation of histotripsy: current status and future directions. Curr Opin Urol 2014;24:104–10.

24. Sukovich J, Xu Z, Kim Y, et al. Targeted Lesion Generation Through the Skull Without Aberration Correction Using Histotripsy. IEEE Trans Ultrason Ferroelectr Freq Control 2016;63:671–82.

25. Sukovich JR, Cain CA, Pandey AS, et al. In vivo histotripsy brain treatment. J Neurosurg 2018;131(4):1331–8.

26. Wu S-K, Santos MA, Marcus SL, et al. MR-guided Focused Ultrasound Facilitates Sonodynamic Therapy with 5-Aminolevulinic Acid in a Rat Glioma Model. Sci Rep 2019;9:10465.

27. Yoshida M, Kobayashi H, Terasaka S, et al. Sonodynamic Therapy for Malignant Glioma Using 220-kHz Transcranial Magnetic Resonance Imaging-Guided Focused Ultrasound and 5-Aminolevulinic acid. Ultrasound Med Biol 2019;45:526–38.

28. Prada F, Sheybani N, Franzini A, et al. Fluorescein-mediated sonodynamic therapy in a rat glioma model. J Neuro Oncol 2020;148:445–54.

29. Zhou Y, Jiao J, Yang R, et al. Temozolomide-based sonodynamic therapy induces immunogenic cell death in glioma. Clin Immunol 2023;256:109772.

30. Mehta NH, Shah HA, D'Amico RS. Sonodynamic Therapy and Sonosensitizers for Glioma Treatment: A Systematic Qualitative Review. World Neurosurg 2023;178:60–8.

31. Hynynen K, McDannold N, Vykhodtseva N, et al. Noninvasive MR imaging-guided focal opening of the blood-brain barrier in rabbits. Radiology 2001;220:640–6.

32. Idbaih A, Canney M, Belin L, et al. Safety and Feasibility of Repeated and Transient Blood-Brain Barrier Disruption by Pulsed Ultrasound in Patients with

Recurrent Glioblastoma. Clin Cancer Res 2019;25:3793–801.

33. Mainprize T, Lipsman N, Huang Y, et al. Blood-Brain Barrier Opening in Primary Brain Tumors with Non-invasive MR-Guided Focused Ultrasound: A Clinical Safety and Feasibility Study. Sci Rep 2019;9:321.

34. Timbie KF, Afzal U, Date A, et al. MR image-guided delivery of cisplatin-loaded brain-penetrating nanoparticles to invasive glioma with focused ultrasound. J Control Release 2017;263:120–31.

35. Fan C-H, Chang E-L, Ting C-Y, et al. Folate-conjugated gene-carrying microbubbles with focused ultrasound for concurrent blood-brain barrier opening and local gene delivery. Biomaterials 2016;106:46–57.

36. Yang Q, Zhou Y, Chen J, et al. Gene Therapy for Drug-Resistant Glioblastoma via Lipid-Polymer Hybrid Nanoparticles Combined with Focused Ultrasound. Int J Nanomed 2021;16:185–99.

37. Pan M, Zhang Y, Deng Z, et al. Noninvasive and Local Delivery of Adenoviral-Mediated Herpes Simplex Virus Thymidine Kinase to Treat Glioma Through Focused Ultrasound-Induced Blood-Brain Barrier Opening in Rats. J Biomed Nanotechnol 2018;14:2031–41.

38. Verhaak RGW, Hoadley KA, Purdom E, et al. Integrated genomic analysis identifies clinically relevant subtypes of glioblastoma characterized by abnormalities in PDGFRA, IDH1, EGFR, and NF1. Cancer Cell 2010;17:98–110.

39. Aldape K, Zadeh G, Mansouri S, et al. Glioblastoma: pathology, molecular mechanisms and markers. Acta Neuropathol 2015;129:829–48.

40. Zhu L, Cheng G, Ye D, et al. Focused Ultrasound-enabled Brain Tumor Liquid Biopsy. Sci Rep 2018;8:6553.

41. Pacia CP, Zhu L, Yang Y, et al. Feasibility and safety of focused ultrasound-enabled liquid biopsy in the brain of a porcine model. Sci Rep 2020;10(1):7449.

42. Sheybani ND, Witter AR, Garrison WJ, et al. Profiling of the immune landscape in murine glioblastoma following blood brain/tumor barrier disruption with MR image-guided focused ultrasound. J Neuro Oncol 2022;156:109–22.

43. Ratnam NM, Gilbert MR, Giles AJ. Immunotherapy in CNS cancers: the role of immune cell trafficking. Neuro Oncol 2019;21:37–46.

44. Vartanian A, Singh SK, Agnihotri S, et al. GBM's multifaceted landscape: highlighting regional and microenvironmental heterogeneity. Neuro Oncol 2014;16:1167–75.

45. Chongsathidkiet P, Jackson C, Koyama S, et al. Sequestration of T cells in bone marrow in the setting of glioblastoma and other intracranial tumors. Nat Med 2018;24:1459–68.

46. Mi Y, Guo N, Luan J, et al. The Emerging Role of Myeloid-Derived Suppressor Cells in the Glioma

Immune Suppressive Microenvironment. Front Immunol 2020;11:737.

47. Vidyarthi A, Agnihotri T, Khan N, et al. Predominance of M2 macrophages in gliomas leads to the suppression of local and systemic immunity. Cancer Immunol Immunother 2019;68:1995–2004.

48. Giles AJ, Hutchinson M-KND, Sonnemann HM, et al. Dexamethasone-induced immunosuppression: mechanisms and implications for immunotherapy. J Immunother Cancer 2018;6:51.

49. Grossman SA, Ye X, Lesser G, et al, NABTT CNS Consortium. Immunosuppression in patients with high-grade gliomas treated with radiation and temozolomide. Clin Cancer Res 2011;17:5473–80.

50. Karachi A, Dastmalchi F, Mitchell DA, et al. Temozolomide for immunomodulation in the treatment of glioblastoma. Neuro Oncol 2018;20:1566–72.

51. Xia J-Z, Xie F-L, Ran L-F, et al. High-intensity focused ultrasound tumor ablation activates autologous tumor-specific cytotoxic T lymphocytes. Ultrasound Med Biol 2012;38:1363–71.

52. Liu F, Hu Z, Qiu L, et al. Boosting high-intensity focused ultrasound-induced anti-tumor immunity using a sparse-scan strategy that can more effectively promote dendritic cell maturation. J Transl Med 2010;8:7.

53. Xing Y, Lu X, Pua EC, et al. The effect of high intensity focused ultrasound treatment on metastases in a murine melanoma model. Biochem Biophys Res Commun 2008;375:645–50.

54. Hu Z, Yang XY, Liu Y, et al. Investigation of HIFU-induced anti-tumor immunity in a murine tumor model. J Transl Med 2007;5:34.

55. Sheybani ND, Batts AJ, Mathew AS, et al. Focused Ultrasound Hyperthermia Augments Release of Glioma-derived Extracellular Vesicles with Differential Immunomodulatory Capacity. Theranostics 2020;10:7436–47.

56. Pellegatta S, Corradino N, Zingarelli M, et al. The Immunomodulatory Effects of Fluorescein-Mediated Sonodynamic Treatment Lead to Systemic and Intratumoral Depletion of Myeloid-Derived Suppressor Cells in a Preclinical Malignant Glioma Model. Cancers 2024;16(4):792.

57. Kovacs ZI, Kim S, Jikaria N, et al. Disrupting the blood-brain barrier by focused ultrasound induces sterile inflammation. Proc Natl Acad Sci USA 2017;114:E75–84.

58. Brighi C, Reid L, White AL, et al. MR-guided focused ultrasound increases antibody delivery to nonenhancing high-grade glioma. Neurooncol Adv 2020;2:vdaa030.

59. Sabbagh A, Beccaria K, Ling X, et al. Opening of the Blood-Brain Barrier Using Low-Intensity Pulsed Ultrasound Enhances Responses to Immunotherapy in Preclinical Glioma Models. Clin Cancer Res 2021;27:4325–37.

60. Chen P-Y, Hsieh H-Y, Huang C-Y, et al. Focused ultrasound-induced blood-brain barrier opening to enhance interleukin-12 delivery for brain tumor immunotherapy: a preclinical feasibility study. J Transl Med 2015;13:93.

Focused Ultrasound for Neurodegenerative Diseases

Rashi I. Mehta, MD[a,b,*], Manish Ranjan, MBBS[c], Marc W. Haut, PhD[b,d,e],
Jeffrey S. Carpenter, MD[a,b,c], Ali R. Rezai, MD[b,c]

KEYWORDS

- Alzheimer's disease • Blood-brain barrier opening • Focused ultrasound
- Magnetic resonance imaging • Neurodegeneration • Neuromodulation • Parkinson's disease

KEY POINTS

- High-intensity focused ultrasound (FUS) ablation is an effective, FDA-approved, and non-invasive surgical treatment option for patients with movement disorder due to essential tremor and Parkinson's disease.
- Blood-brain barrier opening with low-intensity FUS shows promising safety and feasibility in preclinical subjects and clinical trial participants with neurodegeneration and enables noninvasive, targeted intracerebral drug delivery and enhanced drug efficacy.
- Neuromodulation using FUS is an area of active exploration for modification of neurodegenerative disease course.
- Further research and clinical trials are needed to optimize and refine FUS-based techniques to expand treatment options for patients with neurodegenerative diseases.

INTRODUCTION

Neurodegenerative diseases are among the most devastating neurologic disorders and result in damage of neuronal and brain structure.[1,2] These conditions, which predominantly affect the elderly, compromise neurologic function and often culminate in loss of independence and death. Neurodegenerative disorders also pose an overwhelming cost to society and a growing challenge to global healthcare infrastructure.[3]

While progress has been achieved in understanding neurobiology of various neurodegenerative processes,[1,2] disease-modifying therapies remain limited. Uncertainty regarding the precise pathologic mechanisms of these disorders is a hindrance to therapeutic discovery. Furthermore, potentially promising therapies are often confined by their inability to reach diseased brain tissue, due to restrictions imposed by the blood-brain barrier (BBB).[4]

Focused ultrasound (FUS) is an emerging therapeutic option for incurable neurodegenerative conditions.[5] By noninvasive, targeted ultrasonic stimulation of brain tissue, low-intensity FUS (LIFU) causes neuromodulatory effects.[6-9] Upon administration of LIFU energy together with intravenously administered ultrasound contrast agent (microbubbles), secondary neuromodulatory effects are additionally triggered by transient permeabilization of the BBB.[10] This involves enhanced paracellular and transcellular transport

[a] Department of Neuroradiology, Rockefeller Neuroscience Institute, West Virginia University; [b] Department of Neuroscience, Rockefeller Neuroscience Institute, West Virginia University; [c] Department of Neurosurgery, Rockefeller Neuroscience Institute, West Virginia University; [d] Department of Behavioral Medicine and Psychiatry, Rockefeller Neuroscience Institute, West Virginia University; [e] Department of Neurology, Rockefeller Neuroscience Institute, West Virginia University
* Corresponding author. 1 Medical Center Drive, Morgantown, WV 26506.
E-mail address: Rashi.Mehta@hsc.wvu.edu

Magn Reson Imaging Clin N Am 32 (2024) 681–698
https://doi.org/10.1016/j.mric.2024.03.001
1064-9689/24/

and increased cerebral uptake of blood-borne factors.[10] Further, LIFU enables transient BBB disruption for the purpose of targeted intracerebral therapeutic delivery and potentiation of drug efficacy. Focused ultrasound employing high-frequency ultrasound waves (HIFU) offers the ability to modulate brain activity by noninvasively ablating brain targets involved in disordered neural circuitry.[5] Here, the authors review various applications of FUS for the treatment of neurodegenerative diseases and discuss emerging directions in the field.

ALZHEIMER'S DISEASE
Background of Alzheimer's Disease

Alzheimer's disease (AD), the most common neurodegenerative disorder, typically manifests as a chronic progressive multidomain amnestic dementia that ultimately results in disability and death.[3] While the cause of AD is unclear, neuropathological hallmarks of the disease include extracellular β-amyloid deposition and intraneuronal inclusions of tau protein.[11,12] Pathologic and clinical diagnostic consensus guidelines for this disorder have undergone repeated revisions in recent years, highlighting the ambiguity of AD pathophysiology and its clinical definition.[11–14] Nevertheless, it is increasingly clear that AD is a biologically complex disease with evidence of genetic, vascular, and immune contributing factors, among others.[15] While a multitude of hypotheses for AD pathogenesis exist, the amyloid-cascade hypothesis remains a prevailing theory and posits that the intracerebral deposition of β-amyloid is a pivotal initiating event in AD biology.[16] Accordingly, cerebral amyloid aggregates are currently a primary therapeutic target.

Limited treatment options are available for AD.[4,17] Symptomatic treatments including cholinesterase inhibitors and glutamate regulators are widely used but have no significant effect on disease progression.[17] Recently, new immunotherapy drugs have been approved for use in humans by the United States (US) Food and Drug Administration (FDA).[17] Aducanumab and lecanemab, both anti-amyloid monoclonal antibodies, have shown efficacy in reducing β-amyloid plaque load in a dose-dependent manner in individuals with AD.[18,19] Aducanumab, approved through FDA's accelerated approval pathway is being discontinued by the manufacturer.[17] Lecanemab, currently the only traditionally FDA-approved disease-modifying treatment for AD, has shown to slow cognitive decline by 27% after 18 months of use, compared to placebo.[19] However, many patients are ineligible to receive anti-amyloid immunotherapies, which

are known to have potentially serious side effects, including intracerebral hemorrhage, edema, and effusions, that is, amyloid-related imaging abnormalities (ARIA), and infusion reactions.[18–22] Given these limitations and the fact that nearly all biologic drugs are incapable of crossing the BBB,[4] additional disease-modifying therapeutic options and alternative approaches to AD drug delivery are required.[4]

Preclinical Studies of Focused Ultrasound Blood-Brain Barrier Opening in AD Models

Focused ultrasound investigations in animal models of AD have established that BBB opening can be safely achieved under certain parameter conditions that limit erythrocyte extravasation.[23,24] Under such sonication parameters, reconstitution of BBB integrity is shown to occur between 6 and 24 hours in animal models.[24] Beneficial changes in cerebral tissue microenvironment are elicited following single and repeated BBB opening alone (ie, without concurrent therapeutic delivery). This includes reduction of β-amyloid pathology, which has been demonstrated in various AD models and is thought to be an effect of enhanced microglial and astrocytic phagocytosis.[23,25] This hypothesis is supported by histologic evidence of intraparenchymal relocation of endogenous immunoglobulin G (IgG) and immunoglobulin M (IgM) and their colocalization with β-amyloid plaques in the acute phase after BBB opening.[26] Reduction of tau pathology is also documented in various AD animal models and shown to be associated with autophagic mechanisms.[27,28] Works by various teams demonstrate that a sterile inflammatory response is elicited immediately (ie, within the first h[29]) following FUS BBB opening, with various associated transcriptional changes occurring within the first 24 hours.[10,26,29] In addition, trophic factors are recruited to sites of FUS-mediated BBB opening, and are associated with induction of hippocampal neurogenesis and activation of intraneuronal signaling pathways involved in cell survival, growth, and proliferation.[30–32] One study of TgCRND8 mice showed a 250% increase in the number of newborn hippocampal neurons, with increased dendrite length and arborization, 1 month following serial weekly FUS BBB opening procedures.[23] Importantly, FUS BBB opening procedures in various AD models also result in cognitive functional improvements.[10,23]

Additionally, ultrasound-mediated BBB opening facilitates delivery of various therapeutic agents to the brain and is shown to enhance their efficacy. Leininga and colleagues showed that scanning ultrasound increased the delivery of an aducanumab analog (Adu) into brains of APP23 mice, by 5-fold at day 3 following intervention, and resulted in more marked reduction of β-amyloid plaque burden compared to either ultrasound or antibody delivery, alone.[33] This was unassociated with increased rate of cerebral microhemorrhage and was associated with improved spatial memory performance compared to sham-treated APP23 mice, as well as mice treated with antibody alone.[33] Kong and colleagues showed that FUS-mediated BBB opening increased Adu delivery by approximately 8-fold in 5xFAD mice, and this was associated with significantly less cognitive decline and decreased amyloid plaque levels, compared to antibody or FUS treatments, alone.[34] Similarly, BBB opening by FUS enabled delivery of higher concentrations of anti-tau antibodies into brains of pR5 and P301L tau transgenic mice (2 models of tauopathy) and was associated with significantly enhanced efficacy.[35,36] Dubey and colleagues showed that FUS-facilitated intravenous immunoglobulin (IVIg) delivery enhanced reduction of the proinflammatory cytokine TNF-α, which is known to inhibit adult neurogenesis, and promoted hippocampal neurogenesis by 3- and 1.5-fold, relative to IVIg alone or FUS alone, respectively.[37]

Clinical Studies of Focused Ultrasound Blood-Brain Barrier Opening in Alzheimer's Disease

Though few clinical studies have been performed to date, multi-institutional clinical research teams have shown feasibility of FUS-mediated BBB opening in persons with AD. In 2018, a phase 1 trial documented successful BBB opening by FUS with intravenous microbubbles within the targeted subcortical region of the right dorsolateral prefrontal cortex in 5 participants with early to moderate AD.[38] Blood-brain barrier opening was confirmed by MRI detection of gadobutrol contrast extravasation into the targeted zones. This trial study, which used the Insightec 4000 type 2 FUS transducer, showed that the BBB could be safely, reversibly, and repeatedly disrupted with spatial precision and without serious clinical or MRI-evident adverse events.[38] Additionally, there was no clinically significant worsening of cognitive function after targeting non-eloquent region of the frontal lobe in these participants with AD.[38]

Preliminary data from a subsequent ongoing phase 2 trial showed that ultrasound BBB opening was safely performed in the hippocampus and entorhinal cortex of 6 individuals with early AD, without evidence of adverse effects.[39] This multi-institutional FUS study, which also employed the Insightec system, demonstrated the feasibility of

transient BBB disruption within deep intracranial sites and when targeting eloquent cortical brain tissue at regions known to be selectively vulnerable to neurodegeneration by AD.[39] Repeatability of the FUS procedure was also further established in these trial participants, who each underwent three separate BBB opening interventions, administered at 2-week intervals, targeting the medial temporal lobe. Blood-brain barrier closure was verified by MRI evidence of discontinued intraparenchymal gadobutrol contrast extravasation at 24 hours following all procedures. Additional investigation of participants in this phase 2 trial demonstrated the safety and feasibility of FUS BBB opening conducted in more extensive volumes of the brain organ targeting the hippocampus, entorhinal cortex, and frontal and parietal lobes (**Fig. 1**).[40] Safety of multifocal and large-volume BBB opening has also been demonstrated by other clinical trial investigators targeting extensive regions of the frontal lobe parenchyma[41] or multifocal anatomic regions of the default mode network (ie, hippocampus, anterior cingulate gyrus, and precuneus)[42] in patients with AD. Comparison of trial participants' cognitive function to control subjects from the Alzheimer's Disease Neuroimaging Initiative (ADNI) showed no apparent cognitive worsening up to 1 year after FUS treatment.[40,42] Thus, currently available multi-institutional data suggest that BBB opening in multifocal brain sites does not adversely influence AD progression in patients with early disease. Analysis of intracerebral β-amyloid pathology, measured by florbetaben-PET, revealed mild to moderate reductions in plaque load averaging 14% in the centiloid scale in the FUS-treated regions of participants enrolled in our trial.[40] Moderate focal plaque reductions have been detected in various brain regions including the hippocampus and default mode network.[40,42,43]

A limited number of studies have been performed to assess other secondary intracerebral effects of FUS BBB opening in persons with AD.[42,44–46] Interestingly, exploratory investigations of serial post-BBB opening MRI data of our phase 2 trial subjects demonstrated transient alterations in intracerebral fluid flow with permeabilization of downstream veins, consistent with a reactive inflammatory biologic response.[44,45] This transient imaging effect resolved spontaneously within days in all subjects.[44,45] Investigation of resting state functional connectivity in phase 1 trial participants found a transient functional connectivity decrease within the ipsilateral frontoparietal network, following BBB disruption in the right frontal lobe, with recovery of these changes by the following day.[46] No

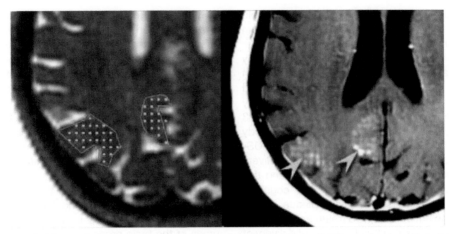

Fig. 1. MRI-guided focused ultrasound-mediated (FUS) blood-brain barrier (BBB) opening in a clinical trial participant with Alzheimer's disease (AD). Target sites (*green dots*) selected by MRI- guidance using T2-weighted sequence in the right parietal lobe of a clinical trial participant with early AD. Spatially precise targeted BBB opening demonstrated on post-contrast T1-weighted image by extravasation of intravenously administered gadobutrol contrast tracer specifically at the targeted zones (*arrowheads*). (*Images reproduced from* Rezai AR et al. Focused ultrasound-mediated blood-brain barrier opening in Alzheimer's disease: long-term safety, imaging, and cognitive outcomes. J Neurosurg. 2022 Nov 4;139(1):275–283, with permission.)

significant differences in resting state connectivity were detected at month 3 comparisons to matched ADNI controls.[46] Analysis of cerebrospinal fluid (CSF) and plasma biomarkers following BBB opening targeting the default mode network did not reveal any significant alteration in CSF AD biomarkers (ie, p-tau181 or amyloid β42/40 ratio) or in biomarkers of BBB dysfunction (ie, plasma platelet-derived growth factor receptor-β (PDGFRβ) and CSF-to-plasma albumin ratio).[42] Yet, more data is needed to further understand these and other MRI and clinical outcomes and potential local and global neuromodulatory effects of this intervention. Moreover, analysis of long-term effects of FUS-mediated BBB opening treatment on Alzheimer's disease course must be studied in larger and more varied human cohorts.

Clinical Studies of Focused Ultrasound Blood-Brain Barrier Opening and Therapeutic Delivery in Alzheimer's Disease

In a recent pilot study, FUS was delivered with each of 6 monthly aducanumab infusions to open the BBB in 3 individuals with early AD.[47] APOE ε4 carriers (homozygotes and heterozygotes) were excluded from participation in this study. Standard aducanumab dose escalation was instituted. Each intervention was well tolerated in all 3 patients, without evidence of serious adverse event attributable to the procedure on cognitive and MRI safety assessments performed over a period of 30 to 180 days after treatment. In each participant, β-amyloid plaque reduction, measured by SUVr and

centiloid scale on serial (18F) florbetaben PET scans, was greater in the FUS-treated areas than in control sites in contralateral homologous brain tissue that was not exposed to FUS (**Fig. 2**).[47] The SUVr reduction in FUS-treated sites averaged 32% for the 3 participants after 26 weeks following completion of the sixth monthly treatment. The degree of β-amyloid reduction was greater than that observed in studies administering FUS alone.[40,43,47] While this study to assess safety and efficacy of FUS-facilitated aducanumab delivery is limited by small sample size, it offers proof-of-concept to support additional investigation of anti-amyloid and therapeutic delivery by FUS in persons with AD and other neurodegenerative diseases. Larger and long-term studies are needed to ensure safety and efficacy of this technique in humans.

Preclinical Studies of Focused Ultrasound Neuromodulation in Alzheimer's Disease Models

Neuromodulation by delivery of LIFU energy alone is currently being investigated in both animal models and humans with neurodegeneration. Advantages of FUS neurostimulation over other modes of neuromodulation include its noninvasiveness, high (millimetric) spatial precision, and ability to selectively target both superficial and deep regions of the brain. The mechanisms of action of this therapy remain uncertain but may be related to direct mechanical effects on membrane and ion channels, mechanosensitive channels, sonoporation, and/or thermal

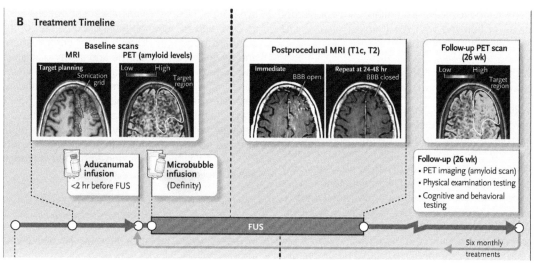

Fig. 2. Outcome summary of a pilot investigation combining focused ultrasound (FUS) and aducanumab in 3 clinical trial participants with Alzheimer's disease (AD). Combined ultrasound blood-brain barrier (BBB) opening and intravenous aducanumab were administered to 3 participants with early AD. Florbetaben PET scan performed 26 weeks following completion of six monthly FUS + Aducanumab treatments showed enhanced amyloid reduction in FUS-treated zones compared to contralateral homologous brain regions not subjected to FUS. (Hynynen, K. Sounding out the Blood–Brain barrier. The New England Journal of Medicine 2024, 390(1), 82-85. https://doi.org/10.1056/nejme2311358.)

effects in addition to possible indirect mechanisms.[48] At present, there is limited preclinical evidence on this technique in AD models, however, available evidence suggest therapeutic effects are promoted by ultrasound neurostimulation. In a study of 5xFAD transgenic mice, LIFU stimulation resulted in improvement of cognitive deficits and significant reduction of cerebral β-amyloid plaque pathology.[49] While the mechanism is unknown, these improved behavioral and proteinopathy effects were associated with increased expression of endothelial nitric oxide synthase (eNOS) and neurotrophic factors and may be related to enhanced cerebral blood flow.[49] Additionally, there was reduced general microgliosis with enhanced recruitment of microglia to β-amyloid deposits, suggesting enhanced plaque phagocytosis.[49] This study also revealed markedly ameliorated cognitive impairments and improved cerebral blood flow, associated with increased eNOS and increased neurogenesis, and oligodendrocytes and remyelination, in a vascular dementia mouse model (bilateral carotid artery stenosis model).[49] In a separate analysis using an aluminum-induced rat model of AD, amyloid concentrations and neuronal damage of the hippocampus were reduced and behavioral deficits were improved.[50] A more recent study assessed effects in a vascular dementia rat model with disease induced by bilateral common carotid artery occlusion (BCCAO).[51] Focused ultrasound sonication to the bilateral medial prefrontal cortex

was performed for 2 weeks after surgery and resulted in significant improvement of working memory task performance, possibly related to improved synaptic function.[51] This was associated with improved cerebral blood flow and reduced neuroinflammation, specifically inhibition of toll-like receptor (TLR4), NF-κB, and decreased proinflammatory cytokines.[51]

Clinical Studies of Focused Ultrasound Neuromodulation in Alzheimer's disease

In an open label clinical study, 22 patients (11 with AD and 11 with Parkinson's disease [PD]) underwent 8 consecutive, weekly focused ultrasound stimulation sessions targeting the hippocampus (AD) or substantia nigra (SNpc) (PD).[52] Sixty-three percent of participants showed improved cognitive exam scores following intervention. Eighty-seven to 88% of patients had stable or improved fine motor and improved gross motor exam scores. No adverse events were encountered. In a subsample of 2 participants, arterial spin labeling (ASL) sequences showed markedly increased perfusion at the targeted hippocampal region after ultrasound stimulation, with greater than 150% increase in relative cerebral blood perfusion at the hippocampi in 1 subject and greater than 50% increase in perfusion in the right hippocampus of the other treated individual.[52] An additional clinical trial study of FUS has recently been initiated to assess potential neuromodulatory effects in humans with AD (ClinicalTrials.gov ID NCT05997030) **(Table 1)**.

PARKINSON'S DISEASE
Background of Parkinson's Disease

Parkinson's disease, the second most common neurodegenerative disorder, typically manifests with bradykinesia, rigidity, tremor, and postural instability. These motor symptoms are associated with degeneration of dopaminergic neurons of the pars compacta region of the substantia nigra (SNpc) and loss of dopaminergic projections in the posterior putamen.[53] On histology, α-synuclein protein inclusions in the SNpc accompanied by neuronal loss confirm the diagnosis.[2] While there is currently no cure for PD, available treatment options include pharmacologic agents (ie, sinemet, primidone, and propranolol), and invasive techniques, such as deep brain stimulation (DBS) and radiofrequency (RF) ablation, for control of motor

symptoms. Neurosurgical treatment options such as DBS and RF ablation have become part of the standard of care in PD with motor complications and have excellent outcome and safety. The invasive nature of neurosurgical therapies, however, deter many patients from choosing effective neurosurgical options, which entail burr holes, brain penetration, and hardware implantation. Gamma knife radiosurgery evolved as a non-invasive ablative treatment in select patients with PD but carries the risk of long-term delayed radiation complications.

Clinical Focused Ultrasound-mediated Neuroablation for Parkinson's Disease

In recent years, ablative therapy via delivery of transcranial HIFU has emerged as an effective non-invasive treatment for select patients with PD and associated motor complication. The FUS ablative technique allows targeting of deep brain structures without the invasiveness of surgery

Table 1
Summary of FUS effects in Alzheimer's disease

FUS Intervention	Outcomes in Preclinical Animal Models	Outcomes in Human Clinical Trial Participants
BBB opening	• Effective BBB permeabilization • No/limited erythrocyte extravasation and edema under certain parameter range • Enhanced delivery of endogenous antibodies into the brain • Microglial and astrocytic activation • Transient sterile inflammation β-amyloid plaque reduction • Intraneural p-tau reduction • Neurogenesis • Activation of Akt (cell survival) signaling • Improved memory performance	• Clinical trials in progress • Effective transient BBB opening • No serious clinical adverse effects • No serious imaging adverse effects • No worsening of cognitive decline (compared to ADNI matched controls) • β-amyloid plaque reduction • Transient alteration of downstream perivenous fluid flow with return to baseline • Transient reduced functional connectivity with return to baseline
BBB opening with therapeutic	• Enhanced delivery of anti-amyloid and anti-tau antibodies • Enhanced delivery of IVIg • Enhanced efficacy of anti-β-amyloid, anti-tau, and IVIg therapies • No evidence of increased microhemorrhage	• Clinical trials in progress • Enhanced effect of intravenously administered aducanumab (greater β-amyloid plaque reduction compared to non-FUS treated regions) • No serious clinical adverse effects • No serious imaging adverse effects
LIFU neuromodulation	• Safe and effective • No intracerebral hemorrhage • Improved cognitive function • Reduced β-amyloid pathology • Improved cerebral blood flow • Reduced microgliosis • Upregulated neurotrophic factors	• Initial clinical trials currently in progress

and with excellent spatial precision. The FDA approved FUS for treatment of tremor-dominant Parkinson's disease in 2018 and subsequently for Parkinson's disease with other motor symptoms such as mobility, rigidity, or dyskinesia symptoms, in 2021 (**Table 2**).

Focused ultrasound ablation for PD entails creation of thermal lesions, by converging high intensity sonication beams, that interrupt neural circuits involved with symptomatic involuntary movements (**Fig. 3**). Ultrasound energy sufficient to cause tissue lesions (ie, 55°C-60°C) is delivered to targeted brain sites and monitored in real time by magnetic resonance thermometry.[54] By convergence of ultrasound energy at a selected focal point in the brain, adverse effects in remaining non-targeted brain parenchyma are limited. Lesioning causes focal necrosis and cytotoxic edema at the targeted site, and expected surrounding vasogenic edema in the acute to subacute period, which is typically maximal at approximately 1 week after FUS treatment (**Fig. 4**).[55] Clinical side effects have been found to peak at 1 week, corresponding to the degree of perilesional edema[56] (**Fig. 4**).

Thalamotomy

For essential tremor and tremor-predominant PD, the nucleus ventralis intermedius (VIM) of the thalamus, which is involved in tremor circuitry that connects the cerebellum with cortical motor pathways, is targeted (see **Fig. 3**). The VIM measures approximately 4 × 4 × 6 mm in size and is not directly visualized by MRI with standard anatomic imaging[57] (see **Fig. 3**). Indirect atlas-based coordinates have been the mainstay of VIM targeting. With empirical/atlas-based methods, targeting is typically performed 15 mm from the midline or 11 mm from the lateral wall of the third ventricle, 1-quarter of the anterior commissure (AC)-posterior commissure (PC) distance anterior to the PC coordinate, using the AC-PC line. The initial indirect AC-PC coordinate is modified based on prior experience and the patient's intraprocedural response. These coordinates serve as a starting point for test sonications that raise target tissue temperatures a few degrees but below cytotoxic levels, akin to the RF temporary ablation. This temporary temperature rise inhibits neural activity and allows assessment of therapeutic response or side effect emergence. Simultaneously, MR thermometry allows confirmation of target location and spot shape characteristics.

It is important to note that unlike conventional stereotactic surgery of DBS and RF thalamotomy, and in addition to lack of discrete visualization of VIM on routine brain MRI sequences, there is no access to electrophysiological localization of the VIM. More direct targeting is feasible using diffusion tractography either primarily or as an adjunct to empirical targeting. This technique can demonstrate the locations of the VIM, pyramidal tract (PT)/internal capsule, and portions of the medial lemniscus (ML)/sensory pathway (see **Fig. 3**). The location of the VIM corresponds to the dentatorubrothalamic tract (DRT) at the z = 0 to 2 mm. The PT/internal capsule and ventral caudalis nucleus of the thalamus are just adjacent to the VIM and are typically located and aid in VIM targeting. One commonly utilized technique of DRT targeting is based on tractography and coregistration with anatomical MRI.[58] The role of DRT and optimal targeting techniques evolved from the experience of DBS.[59] Another technique to target VIM using tractography is to anatomically locate the lateral and posterior borders of the VIM by tracking the PT and ML, respectively.[57] The locations of the sensory thalamus, lemniscus, and PTs were highly precise and were concordant within less than 1 mm between tractography and neurophysiology. A study comparing the treatment locations and potential adverse effect profiles of tractographic VIM targeting with AC-PC based indirect targeting in a larger cohort of FUS thalamotomy suggests that tractographic-based targeting leads to avoidance of areas that are a potential source of adverse effect and result

---

Table 2
Current Food and Drug Administration approved targets for focused ultrasound ablative treatment in Parkinson's disease

Brain Target	Indication	Outcome	Adverse Effect
VIM	Tremor-predominant Parkinson's disease (TD-PD)	Tremor control	Tingling, paresthesia, dysarthria, weakness, loss of taste, and balance disturbance
GPi	Parkinson's disease (PD) with bradykinesia, rigidity, or dyskinesia	Improvement in the bradykinesia, rigidity, or dyskinesia	Tingling, paresthesia, dysarthria, weakness, balance disturbance, loss of taste, and visual field deficit

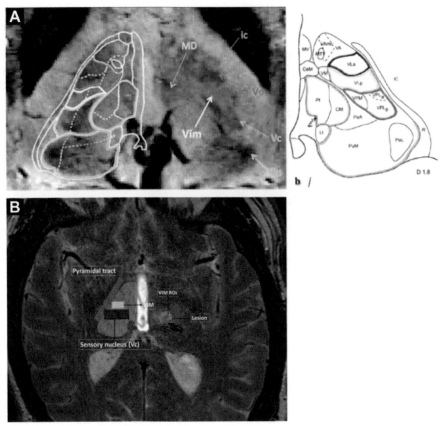

Fig. 3. Ventralis intermedius (VIM) anatomy and targeting. Thalamic nuclei and region of VIM (*yellow arrow*), shown on susceptibility-weighted imaging (SWI) sequence (*A*). The VIM is not discretely discernible on structural MRI. Ventralis intermedius in relation to ventral caudalis (Vc), the sensory nucleus of thalamus (blue), which lies immediately posterior to VIM and pyramidal tract (PT; red), which lies immediately lateral to the VIM (*B*). Tractographic demonstration of PT and medial laminacus (ML) allows localization of internal capsule and Vc respectively, allowing targeting of the VIM 3 mm medial and anterior to these borders, as shown in the left thalamus. ([A] *reproduced from* Najdenovska E et al. Comparison of MRI-based automated segmentation methods and functional neurosurgery targeting with direct visualization of the Ventro-intermediate thalamic nucleus at 7T. Sci Rep. 2019 Feb 4;9(1):1119, with permission. [B] *reproduced from* Krishna V et al. Prospective Tractography-Based Targeting for Improved Safety of Focused Ultrasound Thalamotomy. Neurosurgery. 2019 Jan 1;84(1):160-168, with permission.)

in lesioning more squarely within the VIM.[60] A prospective assessment of tractography-based VIM targeting found that thalamotomy using this guided approach is safe and resulted in no motor or sensory deficits and produced lesions that overlap significantly with VIM defined by probabilistic segmentation.[61]

A prospective multicenter, double-blind randomized, and controlled clinical trial[56] found that unilateral FUS thalamotomy (targeting the VIM) significantly reduced upper extremity tremor scores by 50% at 3 months in patients with moderate-to-severe essential tremor, who were refractory to medical therapy (n = 56), compared to persons who underwent sham procedures (n = 20). Symptomatic improvement was maintained at 12 months following the procedure. Furthermore, measures of disability and quality of life were also improved at 3 months following the treatments. Adverse events following VIM thalamotomy included gait disturbance in 36% of patients and paresthesias or numbness, presumably from lesion involvement of the adjacent ventral posterolateral (sensory) nucleus, in 38%, with these symptoms persisting at 12 months following therapy in 9% to 14% of patients, respectively.[56]

Unilateral FUS thalamotomy is overall well accepted and has a good safety profile. In a safety evaluation assessing 186 patients treated with thalamotomy at 14 centers, severe adverse effects were found to be very infrequent (1%).[62] Most of the encountered side effects were mild and

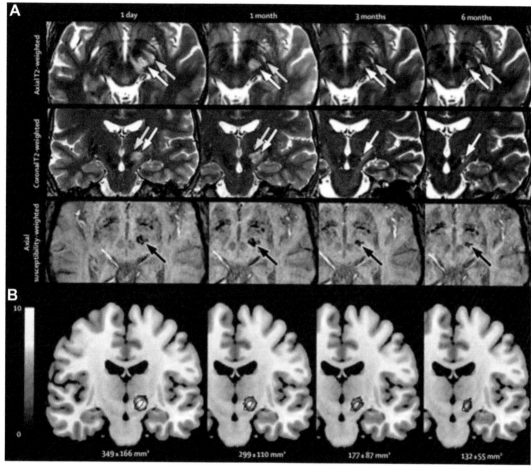

Fig. 4. Temporal MRI effects following unilateral subthalamotomy. Serial T2-weighted and susceptibility-weighted imaging (SWI) images demonstrate edema and hemorrhage at the left subthalamotomy site, decreasing in extent, along with the ablation cavity, over the course of 6 months. (*Reprinted with permission from Elsevier. The Lancet Neurol. 2018 Jan;17(1):54-63.*)

temporary. Sensory abnormality and balance disturbances were the most common FUS thalamotomy related adverse events. A study evaluating the long-term effect of FUS thalamotomy of 45 and 40 patients from a prospective, controlled, multicenter clinical trial who completed follow-up at 4 and 5 years, respectively, reported no new adverse effect and that all previously reported adverse events remained mild or moderate while the therapeutic effect was sustained.[63] The Clinical Rating Scale for Tremor (CRST) and postural tremor scores in the treated hand remained significantly improved by 73% from baseline at 5 years.[63]

Pallidotomy

In 2021, the FDA approved pallidotomy for the treatment of motor complications of PD following a clinical trial assessing FUS pallidotomy in advanced and medically refractory PD.[64]

Anatomically, the globus pallidus internus (GPi) is bound laterally and dorsally by the globus pallidus externa (GPe) and medially by the internal capsule, while ventrally, GPi is in proximity to the optic tracts. The GPi is a relatively large target among the functional neurosurgery targets, and the posteroventrolateral Gpi, its motor territory, is the desired target for PD, especially for PD with dyskinesia. Indirect atlas-based stereotactic coordinates of the GPi are about 19 to 21 mm lateral, 2 to 3 mm anterior, and 4 to 5 mm ventral to the midcommissural point. Unlike the VIM, GPi is discretely visualized on structural MRI brain sequences. The GPi may be directly localized using proton density weighting, SWI/GRE, and FGATIR sequences. Diffusion tractography to delineate and superimpose the internal capsule onto proton density or FGATIR volumetric MRI sequences are particularly useful.

A pivotal open-label trial of unilateral GPi FUS ablation demonstrated a clinically meaningful level of improvement in patients with PD and motor fluctuations, including dyskinesias, with no serious adverse effects.[64] A more recent randomized sham-controlled clinical trial,[65] wherein 94 patients with PD and dyskinesias or motor fluctuations and motor impairment were randomized in a 3:1 ratio to FUS pallidotomy and sham procedures, revealed improved motor function or reduced dyskinesia, however, associated adverse events included dysarthria, gait disturbance, loss of taste, visual disturbance, and facial weakness.[65] A larger trial with long-term followup is necessary to determine the effect and safety of FUS pallidotomy in PD.

Subthalamotomy

The subthalamic nucleus (STN) is the most common target for individuals with PD with motor complication with DBS therapy. The specific target is the dorsolateral (motor) portion of the nucleus. Indirect atlas based stereotactic coordinates are about 11 mm to 13 mm lateral, 3 mm to 4 mm posterior and 4 mm to 5 mm below the midcommissural point. As with the GPi, the STN is directly visualizable to a reasonable degree using high resolution T2, Susceptibility Weighted Imaging (SWI), or Quantitated Susceptibility Mapping (QSM) and MRI can be used to further refine the centroid of the target. Focused ultrasound subthalamotomy has been evaluated in clinical trials and continues to be investigated. In a pilot study of 10 patients with markedly asymmetric parkinsonism that was poorly controlled pharmacologically, FUS subthalamotomy resulted in improvement in the treated hemibody motor status by 53% from baseline to 6 months in the off-medication state and by 47% in the on-medication state.[66] Adverse effects were noted related to subthalamotomy but most were transient. The most frequent adverse events were transient gait ataxia, transient pin-site head pain, and transient high blood pressure. Transient facial asymmetry was noted in 1 patient and moderate impulsivity in 2 patients. A subsequent randomized sham-controlled clinical trial assessed response of poorly-controlled markedly asymmetric patients with PD, who were otherwise not eligible for DBS surgery, to FUS subthalamotomy on the side contralateral to their main motor signs or a sham procedure (2:1 ratio of randomization, respectively).[67] Focused ultrasound subthalamotomy improved motor features of PD in selected patients with asymmetric signs when compared to the sham group with a group difference of 8.1 points in the mean Movement Disorder Society Unified Parkinson's Disease Rating Scale

(MDS-UPDRS) III score. Adverse events included speech and gait disturbances, weakness on the treated side, and dyskinesia, and some of the deficits were persistent at 12 months of reporting.[67] In a recent report of the long-term follow-up of an open label prospective study of 32 patients with asymmetric PD, in which subjects underwent FUS subthalmotomy contralateral to the side of worse motor symptoms, the MDS-UPDRS III score for the treated hemibody off-medication was improved by 52.3% from baseline to 3 years.[68] No disabling or delayed adverse events were reported, but the MDS-UPDRS II, IV, and PDQ39 scores and levodopa dose remained equivalent to those at baseline.

Pallidothalamic tractotomy

Bilateral pallidothalamic tractotomy (PTT) targeting pallidal efferent fibers below the thalamus at the level of Forel's field H1 (either concomitantly or in two sessions) was studied in 10 patients with medically refractory PD.[69] The time frame between baseline UPDRS score and 1 year after the second side was 36 ± 15 months. The total UPDRS score off-medication at 1 year after the second PTT was reduced by 52% compared to that at baseline on-medication. Percentage reductions of the mean scores comparing 1 year off-with baseline on-medication examinations were 91% for tremor, 67% for distal rigidity, and 54% for distal hypobradykinesia. Gait and postural instability were, however, globally unchanged to baseline. Speech difficulties were worsened by 58%. Dyskinesias, dystonia, sleep, and pain were also improved. Mean L-Dopa intake was reduced from 690 ± 250 to 110 ± 190.[69] (Table 3).

Preclinical Studies of Focused Ultrasound Blood-Brain Barrier Opening in Parkinson's Disease Models

Focused ultrasound-mediated BBB opening, to facilitate intracerebral therapeutic delivery and to enhance clearance of protein aggregates, is a promising therapeutic strategy for PD. Various candidate therapeutics such as GDNR, GBA modulators, iron-chelators, antibodies against α-synuclein, and anti-inflammatory factors are all potential options to influence disease course in PD.[70] These FUS studies have shown promising effects in animal models of PD, including restoration of dopaminergic neuron function,[71] decreased α-synuclein in the SNpc and striatum, and reduced microglial activation and inflammation. In one study, adeno-associated virus-glial cell line derived neurotrophic factor (AAV-GDNF) delivery into the left striatum and midbrain of 1-methyl-4-phenyl-1,2,3,6-tetrahydropyridine (MPTP)-treated

Table 3
Current investigational targets for focused ultrasound ablative treatment in Parkinson's disease

Brain Target	Indication	Outcome	Adverse Effect
STN (Unilateral subthalamotomy)	Asymmetric Parkinson's disease with motor complication	Improvement in the tremor and motor symptoms on contralateral side	Dyskinesia (off and on), hemiballismus, speech disturbances, weakness, gait ataxia, impulsivity, and weight increase
PTT (bilateral pallidothalamic tractotomy)	Parkinson's disease with tremor and/or motor complication	Improvement in the tremor and motor symptoms	Hypophonia, speech disturbance, gait disturbance, and anxio-depressive episodes

mice resulted in 58% upregulation of dopaminergic neuronal cell bodies, with 2-fold increase in neuronal projection density.[70] In a separate study, GDNF-liposome-microbubble complexes together with FUS successfully induced BBB opening and improved motor abnormalities in an MPTP-mouse model.[72] Another investigation that combined FUS with nanoparticle delivery, providing GDNF transgene expression in the brain of 6-OHDA-treated rats, resulted in restoration of striatal dopamine levels and dopaminergic neuron density and reversed PD-associated motor dysfunction.[71] In a FUS study of A53T transgenic mice, 3 FUS exposures with anti-α-synuclein antibodies resulted in a 1.5-fold decrease in α-synuclein in the treated hemisphere compared to the untreated brain.[73] An AAV serotype 9 (AAV9) vector bearing a short hairpin RNA sequence targeting the α-synuclein gene was effectively, noninvasively, and simultaneously delivered to multiple brain areas, using FUS, in transgenic mice expressing human α-synuclein.[74]

Clinical Studies of Focused Ultrasound Blood-Brain Barrier Opening in Parkinson's Disease

A limited number of clinical studies show feasibility of BBB opening in humans with PD. A non-randomized phase 1 trial applied 2 successive treatments of FUS with microbubbles to demonstrate safe, reversible, and repeatable BBB opening in the targeted parieto-occipito-temporal cortex of 5 individuals with PD with dementia.[75] A more recent investigation by the same group[76] showed safety and efficacy of BBB opening and delivery of the viral vector AAV9 into nigrostriatal pathways of non-human primates (n = 6) and safety of striatal FUS BBB opening in humans with PD (n = 3). These studies establish a proof-of-concept for future trials in patients with PD, including investigations of gene therapy delivery to targeted brain regions, facilitated by FUS. Recently, in an open-label phase 1 study, investigators demonstrated safety and

feasibility of FUS BBB opening mediated delivery of intravenous lysosomal enzyme glucocerebrosidase (GCase) to the putamen of 4 PD patients with GBA1 mutations.[77] Two patients developed transient dyskinesia after treatment, however, there was no serious adverse effect. Blinded UPDRS motor scores off medication decreased by 12% at 6 months.[77] While prior controlled and randomized clinical trials have established safety and efficacy of gene therapy infusion (eg, gene transfer of glutamic acid decarboxylase into STN[78]) via surgical approach for treatment of patients with PD, the FUS-mediated approach of gene therapy would overcome barriers imposed by invasiveness of intracerebral injections and has potential to address gene expression and permanently modify the disease course.[79] Although very promising, this line of therapeutics requires larger, rigorous, and controlled studies to study and validate safety and efficacy.

Preclinical Studies of Focused Ultrasound Neuromodulation in Parkinson's Disease Models

Recent preclinical studies have shown promising results using low-intensity FUS stimulation in various in vitro and animal PD models.[80] In vitro studies suggest that FUS delivery inhibits MPP+ (1-methyl-4-phenylpyridinium)-induced mitochondrial dysfunction and apoptosis through varied mechanisms. These include decreased mitochondrial reactive oxygen species production, modulation of antioxidant protein expression, prevention of cytochrome C release, and suppression of cleaved-caspase 3 activity.[80–82] In addition, FUS stimulation resulted in decreased MPP+-induced α-synuclein aggregation and levels of phosphorylated α-synuclein.[82] In a mouse model of PD induced by MPTP, FUS stimulation of either the STN or GPi was found to improve motor behavior and to elicit neuroprotective effects, by reducing MPTP toxicity to dopamine neurons.[83] Additional studies in mouse and rat PD models demonstrate restorative effects of FUS stimulation on the nigrostriatal pathway,[84-87] with one study by Xu and colleagues showing increased striatal dopamine levels.[87]

Clinical Studies of Focused Ultrasound Neuromodulation for Parkinson's Disease

Investigations using FUS stimulation in humans are currently limited. In an open label study, 11 patients with PD underwent 8 consecutive and weekly focused ultrasound stimulation sessions targeting the SNpc (PD) and showed stable or improved fine motor and gross motor exam scores.[52] A recent randomized sham-controlled study examined the feasibility of bilateral primary motor cortex stimulation with theta-burst FUS in 10 patients with PD and found that FUS application increases motor cortex excitability and is thus a feasible noninvasive neuromodulation strategy in PD.[88] Larger longitudinal studies are needed to further evaluate clinical effects and optimal protocols using this technique for PD in humans (Table 4).

AMYOTROPHIC LATERAL SCLEROSIS
Background of Amyotrophic Lateral Sclerosis

Among the neurodegenerative disorders, amyotrophic lateral sclerosis (ALS) is the third most common and the most rapidly fatal.[89] This debilitating disease results in selective degeneration of motor neurons of the brain, brainstem, and spinal cord.[89,90] Amyotrophic lateral sclerosis causes insidious denervation of voluntary muscles and progressive functional disability. Death typically ensues, within 2 years to 3 years of symptom onset, secondary to neuromuscular respiratory failure.[89] Approximately 5% of patients with ALS develop clinically overt frontotemporal dementia (FTD), however, this statistic underrepresents the actual degree of overlap between the 2 disorders, which are now considered entities of a single disease continuum.[89,91] TAR DNA-binding protein 43 (TDP-43) accumulation is observed in most cases, and overlaps with neuropathologic change of other neurodegenerative processes, including FTD.[2] Familial ALS with various modes of inheritance is believed to be responsible for 10% to 15% of cases.

Considerable pathologic heterogeneity of ALS has been well documented, with over 40 genes found to be associated with this disorder.[92,93] Of these, 4 genetic abnormalities account for approximately half of familial cases and approximately 5% of sporadic cases.[92,93] Greater than 60 candidate therapies with diverse mechanisms of action have been investigated in clinical trials for ALS.[89] Few therapeutics, however, have been approved for clinical use to slow progression or improve

Table 4
Investigational low-intensity focused ultrasound outcomes in Parkinson's disease

FUS Intervention	Outcomes in Preclinical Animal Models	Outcomes in Human Clinical Trial Participants
BBB opening/Therapeutic delivery	• Reduced neuroinflammation • Decreased α-synuclein in SNpc/striatum • Restoration of dopamine neuron function • Improved motor abnormalities	• Safe, effective, reversible, and repeatable BBB opening • Delivery of glucocerebrosidase in putamen • No serious adverse effects • Improved motor function
LIFU neuromodulation	• Improved motor behavior • Protection against MPTP-induced neurotoxicity in dopaminergic neurons • Reduced 6-OHDA-induced neurotoxicity • Increased striatal superoxide dismutase • Increased dopamine in the striatum • Increased number of TH neurons in the SNpc • Increased levels of GDNF in the SNpc • Reduced neuroinflammation • Decreased apoptosis in SNpc • No tissue damage or cytotoxicity	• Stable/improved fine/gross motor exam stores • Increased motor cortex excitability

symptomatology of ALS.[94] These include Riluzole, a glutamate blocker that reduces excitotoxicity; edaravone, an antioxidant that protects neurons from damaging effects of reactive oxygen species; and AMX0035, which targets mitochondrial and endoplasmic reticulum cell death pathways.[94] Toferson, an antisense oligonucleotide that targets the production of superoxide dismutase 1, was also approved by the FDA in 2023.[94] Current ALS therapies have limited benefits, with prolongation of survival on the order of months.[89]

Preclinical Studies of Focused Ultrasound in Amyotrophic Lateral Sclerosis Models

Animal studies have reported beneficial effects following surgical injection of various therapeutic agents, including AAV encoding short hairpin RNA and neural progenitor cells, into the brain motor cortex. Limited preclinical data exist on the use of FUS for ALS. A recent study aimed to facilitate edaravone delivery into brain in a transgenic mouse model of ALS.[95] In this investigation, BBB opening by FUS was found to enhance delivery, by 2-fold, of edaravone to the targeted motor cortex of SOD1^{G93A} mice, without evidence of tissue injury.[95] Moreover, ultrasound-enhanced delivery of edaravone was shown to provide additive improvement on disease progression. Specifically, mice treated by FUS-enhanced edaravone delivery exhibited improvements in neuromuscular functions (ie, gait, muscle strength, and motor coordination) relative to mice treated with edaravone alone. Improved rescue of muscle atrophy was demonstrated in the FUS-treated mice. In addition, neuroprotective effects were found to occur in both upper and lower motor neurons as indicated by normalized neuronal morphology (ie, increasing cell body size), and significant alleviation of neuroinflammation and misfolded SOD1 protein, were shown on histologic examination in

mice treated with FUS-enhanced edaravone delivery.[95] While this study shows promising effects, the SOD1^{G93A} mouse model does not fully recapitulate pathologic effects of ALS in humans, including TDP-43 and additional heterogeneous pathology, and much additional preclinical and clinical work is needed to evaluate efficacy of FUS-enhanced drug delivery in ALS. (Table 5).

Clinical Studies of Focused Ultrasound Blood-Brain Barrier Opening in Amyotrophic Lateral Sclerosis

An initial report of a phase 1 trial documents safety and efficacy of FUS BBB opening in 4 individuals with ALS.[96] In this study, the primary motor cortex was treated, using motor task fMRI to localize and target functional arm and leg-controlling sites. This study shows that the BBB of the eloquent motor cortex and subcortical tissue can be reversibly permeabilized by ultrasound without serious adverse effects in persons with ALS. This ongoing study sets the stage for future trials that will evaluate safety and efficacy of FUS-mediated therapeutic delivery to areas of neurodegeneration in ALS. Preclinical studies have shown prolonged survival following infusion of AAVs, antibodies (ie, against SOD1), and progenitor cells, delivered by invasive surgical technique, in ALS animal models. As mutations associated with ALS are amenable to gene-based therapies,[90,92] FUS-facilitated gene therapy will be an important and potentially transformative area of future investigation.[97] Genetic profiling is expected to play a critical role in patient selection for future gene-based precision-approach therapies for ALS cases attributable to genetic etiologies.[90,92]

FUTURE DIRECTIONS AND CONCLUSION

Over recent years, the feasibility of various clinical FUS applications has been established. Additional

Table 5
Investigational low-intensity focused ultrasound outcomes in amyotrophic lateral sclerosis

FUS Intervention	Outcomes in Preclinical Animal Models	Outcomes in Human Clinical Trial Participants
BBB opening/Therapeutic delivery	• Enhanced delivery of edaravone (2x) • No evidence of tissue injury • Additive improvement on disease progression (improvements in gait, muscle strength, and motor coordination) • Improved rescue of muscle atrophy • Neuroprotective effects (increasing cell body size, decreased neuroinflammation, and decreased misfolded SOD1 protein)	• Safe and effective BBB opening

work is needed to clarify underlying mechanisms of action and to fine-tune procedural techniques to maximize efficacy and safety of varied clinical FUS procedures. Next steps include expanded clinical trial investigations employing standardized methods and outcome measures to clarify optimal ultrasound parameters and study protocols in larger sample populations.[98] Moreover, studies in diverse cohorts are needed to understand effects of FUS procedures in persons across race, sex, age, and disease stage. Understanding how these factors as well as genetic and comorbid diseases influence outcomes will be important for defining ideal patient inclusion and exclusion criteria for specific FUS treatments. In parallel with this, systematic MRI investigations are needed to identify and validate appropriate short-term and long-term imaging biomarkers to gauge efficacy and clinical responses to FUS interventions. Progress in these areas will aid in development of personalized approaches using FUS technologies and leverage new drugs and gene therapies, with disease modifying potential[97,99], for persons with AD, PD, ALS, Huntington's disease, and other forms of neurodegeneration.

CLINICS CARE POINTS

- MRI plays a critical role in optimal brain targeting for various FUS techniques.
- MRI demonstrates typical evolutionary changes at sites of FUS neuroablation, with perilesional edema maximizing at approximately one week post intervention and gradual retraction of the necrotic ablation cavity.
- MRI investigations reveal neuromodulatory effects of FUS stimulation and FUS-mediated BBB opening, although additional work is needed to further understand these responses in humans.
- FUS-facilitated aducanumab delivery results in enhanced amyloid plaque reduction, as measured by (18F) florbetaben PET.

DISCLOSURE

The authors have no relevant disclosures.

REFERENCES

1. Dugger BN, Dickson DW. Pathology of neurodegenerative diseases. Cold Spring Harb Perspect Biol 2017;9(7):a028035.
2. Mehta RI, Schneider JA. Neuropathology of the common forms of dementia. Clin Geriatr Med 2023;39(1):91–107.
3. Alzheimer's Association. 2023 Alzheimer's disease facts and figures. Alzheimers Dement 2023;19(4). https://doi.org/10.1002/alz.13016.
4. Pardridge WM. Treatment of Alzheimer's disease and blood-brain barrier drug delivery. Pharmaceuticals (Basel) 2020;13(11):394.
5. Krishna V, Sammartino F, Rezai A. A review of the current therapies, challenges, and future directions of transcranial focused ultrasound technology: advances in diagnosis and treatment. JAMA Neurol 2018;75(2):246–54.
6. Badran BW, Caulfield KA, Stomberg-Firestein S, et al. Sonication of the anterior thalamus with MRI-Guided transcranial focused ultrasound (tFUS) alters pain thresholds in healthy adults: A double-blind, sham-controlled study. Brain Stimul 2020;13(6):1805–12.
7. Leo Ai, Mueller JK, Grant A, et al. Transcranial focused ultrasound for BOLD fMRI signal modulation in humans. Annu Int Conf IEEE Eng Med Biol Soc 2016;1758–61.
8. Mahoney JJ, Haut MW, Carpenter J, et al. Low-intensity focused ultrasound targeting the nucleus accumbens as a potential treatment for substance use disorder: safety and feasibility clinical trial. Front Psychiatry 2023;14:1211566.
9. Mahoney JJ 3rd, Hanlon CA, Marshalek PJ, et al. Transcranial magnetic stimulation, deep brain stimulation, and other forms of neuromodulation for substance use disorders: Review of modalities and implications for treatment. J Neurol Sci 2020;418:117149.
10. Todd N, Angolano C, Ferran C, et al. Secondary effects on brain physiology caused by focused ultrasound-mediated disruption of the blood-brain barrier. J Contr Release 2020;324:450–9.
11. Jack CR Jr, Bennett DA, Blennow K, et al. Contributors. NIA-AA research framework: toward a biological definition of Alzheimer's disease. Alzheimers Dement 2018;14(4):535–62.
12. Mehta RI, Schneider JA. What is 'Alzheimer's disease'? The neuropathological heterogeneity of clinically defined Alzheimer's dementia. Curr Opin Neurol 2021;34(2):237–45.
13. Jack CR, et al. Revised criteria for diagnosis and staging of Alzheimer's Disease: Alzheimer's Association Workgroup. In Alzheimer's Association International Conference. 2024. Available at: https://aaic.alz.org/diagnostic-criteria.asp. [Accessed 14 February 2024].
14. McKhann GM, Knopman DS, Chertkow H, et al. The diagnosis of dementia due to Alzheimer's disease: recommendations from the National Institute on Aging-Alzheimer's Association workgroups on

diagnostic guidelines for Alzheimer's disease. Alzheimers Dement 2011;7(3):263–9.

15. Mehta RI, Mehta RI. The vascular-immune hypothesis of Alzheimer's Disease. Biomedicines 2023; 11(2):408.

16. Hardy J, Selkoe DJ. The amyloid hypothesis of Alzheimer's disease: progress and problems on the road to therapeutics. Science 2002;297(5580):353–6.

17. Alzheimer's Association. Medications for memory, cognition and dementia-Related Behaviors. 2024. Available at: https://www.alz.org/alzheimers-dementia/treatments/medications-for-memory. [Accessed 14 February 2024].

18. Budd Haeberlein S, Aisen PS, Barkhof F, et al. Two randomized phase 3 studies of aducanumab in early Alzheimer's disease. J Prev Alzheimers Dis 2022;9:197–210.

19. van Dyck CH, Swanson CJ, Aisen P, et al. Lecanemab in early Alzheimer's disease. N Engl J Med 2023;388. 9-2.

20. Cummings J, Aisen P, Apostolova LG, et al. Aducanumab: appropriate use recommendations. J Prev Alzheimers Dis 2021;8(4):398–410.

21. Cummings J, Rabinovici GD, Atri A, et al. Aducanumab: appropriate use recommendations update. J Prev Alzheimers Dis 2022;9(2):221–30.

22. Sperling RA, Jack CR Jr, Black SE, et al. Amyloid-related imaging abnormalities in amyloid-modifying therapeutic trials: recommendations from the Alzheimer's Association Research Roundtable Workgroup. Alzheimers Dement 2011;7(4):367–85.

23. Burgess A, Dubey S, Yeung S, et al. Alzheimer disease in a mouse model: MR imaging-guided focused ultrasound targeted to the hippocampus opens the blood-brain barrier and improves pathologic abnormalities and behavior. Radiology 2014; 273(3):736–45.

24. Meng Y, Pople CB, Lea-Banks H, et al. Safety and efficacy of focused ultrasound induced blood-brain barrier opening, an integrative review of animal and human studies. J Contr Release 2019;309:25–36.

25. Leinenga G, Götz J. Scanning ultrasound removes amyloid-β and restores memory in an Alzheimer's disease mouse model. Sci Transl Med 2015; 7(278). 278ra233.

26. Jordão JF, Thévenot E, Markham-Coultes K, et al. Amyloid-β plaque reduction, endogenous antibody delivery and glial activation by brain-targeted, transcranial focused ultrasound. Exp Neurol 2013;248:16–29.

27. Pandit R, Leinenga G, Götz J. Repeated ultrasound treatment of tau transgenic mice clears neuronal tau by autophagy and improves behavioral functions. Theranostics 2019;9(13):3754–67.

28. Karakatsani ME, Kugelman T, Ji R, et al. Unilateral focused ultrasound-induced blood-brain barrier opening reduces phosphorylated Tau from The rTg4510 mouse model. Theranostics 2019;9(18):5396–411.

29. Kovacs ZI, Kim S, Jikaria N, et al. Disrupting the blood-brain barrier by focused ultrasound induces sterile inflammation. Proc Natl Acad Sci U S A 2017;114(1):E75–84.

30. Jalali S, Huang Y, Dumont DJ, et al. Focused ultrasound-mediated bbb disruption is associated with an increase in activation of AKT: experimental study in rats. BMC Neurol 2010;10:114.

31. Scarcelli T, Jordão JF, O'Reilly MA, et al. Stimulation of hippocampal neurogenesis by transcranial focused ultrasound and microbubbles in adult mice. Brain Stimul 2014;7(2):304–7.

32. Shin J, Kong C, Lee J, et al. Focused ultrasound-induced blood-brain barrier opening improves adult hippocampal neurogenesis and cognitive function in a cholinergic degeneration dementia rat model. Alzheimer's Res Ther 2019;11(1):110.

33. Leinenga G, Koh WK, Götz J. A comparative study of the effects of Aducanumab and scanning ultrasound on amyloid plaques and behavior in the APP23 mouse model of Alzheimer disease. Alzheimer's Res Ther 2021;13(1):76.

34. Kong C, Yang EJ, Shin J, et al. Enhanced delivery of a low dose of aducanumab via FUS in 5×FAD mice, an AD model. Transl Neurodegener 2022; 11(1):57.

35. Janowicz PW, Leinenga G, Götz J, et al. Ultrasound-mediated blood-brain barrier opening enhances delivery of therapeutically relevant formats of a tau-specific antibody. Sci Rep 2019;9(1):9255.

36. Nisbet RM, Van der Jeugd A, Leinenga G, et al. Combined effects of scanning ultrasound and a tau-specific single chain antibody in a tau transgenic mouse model. Brain 2017;140(5):1220–30.

37. Dubey S, Heinen S, Krantic S, et al. Clinically approved IVIg delivered to the hippocampus with focused ultrasound promotes neurogenesis in a model of Alzheimer's disease. Proc Natl Acad Sci U S A 2020;117(51):32691–700.

38. Lipsman N, Meng Y, Bethune AJ, et al. Blood-brain barrier opening in Alzheimer's disease using MR-guided focused ultrasound. Nat Commun 2018; 9(1):2336.

39. Rezai AR, Ranjan M, D'Haese PF, et al. Noninvasive hippocampal blood-brain barrier opening in Alzheimer's disease with focused ultrasound. Proc Natl Acad Sci U S A 2020;117(17):9180–2.

40. Rezai AR, Ranjan M, Haut MW, Alzheimer's Disease Neuroimaging Initiative. Focused ultrasound-mediated blood-brain barrier opening in Alzheimer's disease: long-term safety, imaging, and cognitive outcomes. J Neurosurg 2022;139(1):275–83.

41. Park SH, Baik K, Jeon S, et al. Extensive frontal focused ultrasound mediated blood-brain barrier opening for the treatment of Alzheimer's disease: a proof-of-concept study. Transl Neurodegener 2021; 10(1):44.

42. Meng Y, Goubran M, Rabin JS, et al. Blood-brain barrier opening of the default mode network in Alzheimer's disease with magnetic resonance-guided focused ultrasound. Brain 2023;146(3):865–72.

43. D'Haese PF, Ranjan M, Song A, et al. β-Amyloid Plaque Reduction in the Hippocampus After Focused Ultrasound-Induced Blood-Brain Barrier Opening in Alzheimer's Disease. Front Hum Neurosci 2020;14: 593672.

44. Mehta RI, Carpenter JS, Mehta RI, et al. Blood-Brain Barrier Opening with MRI-guided Focused Ultrasound Elicits Meningeal Venous Permeability in Humans with Early Alzheimer Disease. Radiology 2021;298(3):654–62.

45. Mehta RI, Carpenter JS, Mehta RI, et al. Ultrasound-mediated blood-brain barrier opening uncovers an intracerebral perivenous fluid network in persons with Alzheimer's disease. Fluids Barriers CNS 2023;20(1):46.

46. Meng Y, MacIntosh BJ, Shirzadi Z, et al. Resting state functional connectivity changes after MR-guided focused ultrasound mediated blood-brain barrier opening in patients with Alzheimer's disease. Neuroimage 2019;200:275–80.

47. Rezai AR, D'Haese PF, Finomore V, et al. Ultrasound Blood-Brain Barrier Opening and Aducanumab in Alzheimer's Disease. N Engl J Med 2024;390(1): 55–62.

48. Pople CB, Meng Y, Li DZ, et al. Neuromodulation in the Treatment of Alzheimer's Disease: Current and Emerging Approaches. J Alzheimers Dis 2020; 78(4):1299–313.

49. Eguchi K, Shindo T, Ito K, et al. Whole-brain low-intensity pulsed ultrasound therapy markedly improves cognitive dysfunctions in mouse models of dementia - Crucial roles of endothelial nitric oxide synthase. Brain Stimul 2018;11(5):959–73.

50. Lin WT, Chen RC, Lu WW, et al. Protective effects of low-intensity pulsed ultrasound on aluminum-induced cerebral damage in Alzheimer's disease rat model. Sci Rep 2015;5:9671.

51. Wang F, Wang Q, Wang L, et al. Low-Intensity Focused Ultrasound Stimulation Ameliorates Working Memory Dysfunctions in Vascular Dementia Rats via Improving Neuronal Environment. Front Aging Neurosci 2022;14:814560.

52. Nicodemus NE, Becerra S, Kuhn TP, et al. Focused transcranial ultrasound for treatment of neurodegenerative dementia. Alzheimers Dement (N Y) 2019;5: 374–81.

53. Surmeier DJ, Obeso JA, Halliday GM. Selective neuronal vulnerability in Parkinson disease. Nat Rev Neurosci 2017;18(2):101–13.

54. Mattay RR, Kim K, Shah L, et al. MR Thermometry during Transcranial MR Imaging-Guided Focused Ultrasound Procedures: A Review. AJNR Am J Neuroradiol 2023;45(1):1–8.

55. Blitz SE, Torre M. Chua MMJ, et al. Focused Ultrasound Thalamotomy: Correlation of Postoperative Imaging with Neuropathological Findings. Stereotact Funct Neurosurg 2023;101(1):60–7.

56. Elias WJ, Lipsman N, Ondo WG, et al. A Randomized Trial of Focused Ultrasound Thalamotomy for Essential Tremor. N Engl J Med 2016;375(8):730–9.

57. Sammartino F, Krishna V, King NK, et al. Tractography-Based Ventral Intermediate Nucleus Targeting: Novel Methodology and Intraoperative Validation. Mov Disord 2016;31(8):1217–25.

58. Chazen JL, Sarva H, Stieg PE, et al. Clinical improvement associated with targeted interruption of the cerebellothalamic tract following MR-guided focused ultrasound for essential tremor. J Neurosurg 2018; 129(2):315–23.

59. Coenen VA, Allert N, Mädler B. A role of diffusion tensor imaging fiber tracking in deep brain stimulation surgery: DBS of the dentato-rubro-thalamic tract (drt) for the treatment of therapy-refractory tremor. Acta Neurochir 2011;153(8):1579–85 [discussion 1585].

60. Ranjan M, Elias GJB, Boutet A, et al. Tractography-based targeting of the ventral intermediate nucleus: accuracy and clinical utility in MRgFUS thalamotomy. J Neurosurg 2019;1–8.

61. Krishna V, Sammartino F, Agrawal P, et al. Prospective Tractography-Based Targeting for Improved Safety of Focused Ultrasound Thalamotomy. Neurosurgery 2019;84(1):160–8.

62. Fishman PS, Elias WJ, Ghanouni P, et al. Neurological adverse event profile of magnetic resonance imaging-guided focused ultrasound thalamotomy for essential tremor. Mov Disord 2018;33(5):843–7.

63. Cosgrove GR, Lipsman N, Lozano AM, et al. Magnetic resonance imaging-guided focused ultrasound thalamotomy for essential tremor: 5-year follow-up results. J Neurosurg 2022;138(4):1028–33.

64. Eisenberg HM, Krishna V, Elias WJ, et al. MR-guided focused ultrasound pallidotomy for Parkinson's disease: safety and feasibility. J Neurosurg 2020; 135(3):792–8.

65. Krishna V, Fishman PS, Eisenberg HM, et al. Trial of Globus Pallidus Focused Ultrasound Ablation in Parkinson's Disease. N Engl J Med 2023;388(8):683–93.

66. Martínez-Fernández R, Rodríguez-Rojas R, Del Álamo M, et al. Focused ultrasound subthalamotomy in patients with asymmetric Parkinson's disease: a pilot study. Lancet Neurol 2018;17(1):54–63.

67. Martínez-Fernández R, Máñez-Miró JU, Rodríguez-Rojas R, et al. Randomized Trial of Focused Ultrasound Subthalamotomy for Parkinson's Disease. N Engl J Med 2020;383(26):2501–13.

68. Martínez-Fernández R, Natera-Villalba E, Máñez Miró JU, et al. Prospective Long-term Follow-up of Focused Ultrasound Unilateral Subthalamotomy for Parkinson Disease. Neurology 2023;100(13): e1395–405.

69. Gallay MN, Moser D, Magara AE, et al. Bilateral MR-Guided Focused Ultrasound Pallidothalamic Tractotomy for Parkinson's Disease With 1-Year Follow-Up. Front Neurol 2021;12:601153.

70. Karakatsani ME, Blesa J, Konofagou EE. Blood-brain barrier opening with focused ultrasound in experimental models of Parkinson's disease. Mov Disord 2019;34(9):1252–61.

71. Mead BP, Kim N, Miller GW, et al. Novel Focused Ultrasound Gene Therapy Approach Noninvasively Restores Dopaminergic Neuron Function in a Rat Parkinson's Disease Model. Nano Lett 2017;17(6):3533–42.

72. Lin CY, Hsieh HY, Chen CM, et al. Non-invasive, neuron-specific gene therapy by focused ultrasound-induced blood-brain barrier opening in Parkinson's disease mouse model. J Contr Release 2016;235:72–81.

73. Zhang H, Sierra C, Kwon N, et al. Focused-ultrasound Mediated Anti-Alpha-Synuclein Antibody Delivery for the Treatment of Parkinson's Disease. In: IEEE International ultrasonics Symposium, IUS, 22-25 October. Kobe, Japan; 2018.

74. Xhima K, Nabbouh F, Hynynen K, et al. Noninvasive delivery of an α-synuclein gene silencing vector with magnetic resonance-guided focused ultrasound. Mov Disord 2018;33(10):1567–79.

75. Gasca-Salas C, Fernández-Rodríguez B, Pineda-Pardo JA, et al. Blood-brain barrier opening with focused ultrasound in Parkinson's disease dementia. Nat Commun 2021;12(1):779.

76. Blesa J, Pineda-Pardo JA, Inoue KI, et al. BBB opening with focused ultrasound in nonhuman primates and Parkinson's disease patients: Targeted AAV vector delivery and PET imaging. Sci Adv 2023;9(16):eadf4888.

77. Meng Y, Pople CB, Huang Y, et al. Putaminal Recombinant Glucocerebrosidase Delivery with Magnetic Resonance-Guided Focused Ultrasound in Parkinson's Disease: A Phase I Study. Mov Disord 2022;37(10):2134–9.

78. LeWitt PA, Rezai AR, Leehey MA, et al. AAV2-GAD gene therapy for advanced Parkinson's disease: a double-blind, sham-surgery controlled, randomised trial. Lancet Neurol 2011;10(4):309–19.

79. Fan C-H, Lin C-Y, Liu H-L, et al. Ultrasound targeted CNS gene delivery for Parkinson's disease treatment. J Contr Release 2017;261:246–62.

80. Lee KS, Clennell B, Steward TGJ, et al. Focused Ultrasound Stimulation as a Neuromodulatory Tool for Parkinson's Disease: A Scoping Review. Brain Sci 2022;12(2):289.

81. Zhao L, Feng Y, Shi A, et al. Neuroprotective Effect of Low-Intensity Pulsed Ultrasound Against MPP+-Induced Neurotoxicity in PC12 Cells: Involvement of K2P Channels and Stretch-Activated Ion Channels. Ultrasound Med Biol 2017;43(9):1986–99.

82. Karmacharya MB, Hada B, Park SR, et al. Low-Intensity Ultrasound Decreases α-Synuclein Aggregation via Attenuation of Mitochondrial Reactive Oxygen Species in MPP(+)-Treated PC12 Cells. Mol Neurobiol 2017;54(8):6235–44.

83. Zhou H, Niu L, Meng L, et al. Noninvasive Ultrasound Deep Brain Stimulation for the Treatment of Parkinson's Disease Model Mouse. Research 2019;1748489.

84. Chen X, Wang D, Zhang L, et al. Neuroprotective Effect of Low-Intensity Pulsed Ultrasound on the Mouse MPTP/MPP+ Model of Dopaminergic Neuron Injury. Ultrasound Med Biol 2021;47(8):2321–30.

85. Dong Y, Liu D, Zhao Y, et al. Assessment of Neuroprotective Effects of Low-Intensity Transcranial Ultrasound Stimulation in a Parkinson's Disease Rat Model by Fractional Anisotropy and Relaxation Time T2* Value. Front Neurosci 2021;15:590354.

86. Sung CY, Chiang PK, Tsai CW, et al. Low-Intensity Pulsed Ultrasound Enhances Neurotrophic Factors and Alleviates Neuroinflammation in a Rat Model of Parkinson's Disease. Cerebr Cortex 2021;32(1):176–85.

87. Xu T, Lu X, Peng D, et al. Ultrasonic stimulation of the brain to enhance the release of dopamine - A potential novel treatment for Parkinson's disease. Ultrason Sonochem 2020;63:104955.

88. Samuel N, Ding MYR, Sarica C, et al. Accelerated Transcranial Ultrasound Neuromodulation in Parkinson's Disease: A Pilot Study. Mov Disord 2023;38(12):2209–16.

89. Mead RJ, Shan N, Reiser HJ, et al. Amyotrophic lateral sclerosis: a neurodegenerative disorder poised for successful therapeutic translation. Nat Rev Drug Discov 2023;22(3):185–212.

90. Goutman SA, Hardiman O, Al-Chalabi A, et al. Emerging insights into the complex genetics and pathophysiology of amyotrophic lateral sclerosis. Lancet Neurol 2022;21(5):465–79.

91. Burrell JR, Halliday GM, Kril JJ, et al. The frontotemporal dementia-motor neuron disease continuum. Lancet 2016;388(10047):919–31.

92. Goutman SA, Hardiman O, Al-Chalabi A, et al. Recent advances in the diagnosis and prognosis of amyotrophic lateral sclerosis. Lancet Neurol 2022;21(5):480–93.

93. Zou ZY, Zhou ZR, Che CH, et al. Genetic epidemiology of amyotrophic lateral sclerosis: a systematic review and meta-analysis. J Neurol Neurosurg Psychiatry 2017;88(7):540–9.

94. ALS Association. FDA-Approved Drugs for Treating ALS. 2024. Available at: https://www.als.org/navigating-als/living-with-als/fda-approved-drugs. [Accessed 14 February 2024].

95. Shen Y, Zhang J, Xu Y, et al. Ultrasound-enhanced brain delivery of edaravone provides additive amelioration on disease progression in an ALS mouse model. Brain Stimul 2023;16(2):628–41.

96. Abrahao A, Meng Y, Llinas M, et al. First-in-human trial of blood-brain barrier opening in amyotrophic lateral sclerosis using MR-guided focused ultrasound. Nat Commun 2019;10(1):4373.

97. Kofoed RH, Aubert I. Focused ultrasound gene delivery for the treatment of neurological disorders. Trends Mol Med 2024;30(3):263–77.

98. Focused Ultrasound Foundation, Focused Ultrasound for Alzheimer's Disease Workshop [White paper], Available at: https://cdn.fusfoundation.org/2023/08/28125240/2023-FUSF-Alzheimers-Disease-Workshop-Summary.pdf, (Accessed 14 February 2024), 2023.

99. Hynynen K. Sounding Out the Blood-Brain Barrier. N Engl J Med 2024 Jan 4;390(1):82–5.

The Use of Focused Ultrasound to Enhance Liquid Biopsy

Ying Meng, MD[a,b], Christopher B. Pople, MSc[b], Nir Lipsman, MD, PhD[a,b],*

KEYWORDS

• Focused ultrasound • Blood–brain barrier disruption • Liquid biopsy

KEY POINTS

• Focused ultrasound liquid biopsy is an emerging area of research in liberating biomarkers in the brain by temporary disruption of the blood–brain barrier.
• This approach promises to provide spatial selectivity that cannot be achieved with liquid biopsy alone.
• This field is in its infancy and more data through collaborative efforts between various stakeholders and users will be needed to develop its applications.
• The development of focused ultrasound technology is headed toward better integration into clinical care pathways, lessening the burden for patients.

INTRODUCTION

Breakthroughs in medical imaging and ultrasound transducer design have led to feasible application of focused ultrasound (FUS) to intracranial pathologies.[1] These technologies have allowed FUS to be delivered more precisely and accurately. At present, the only clinically approved therapeutic use of FUS is the thermal ablation of deep targets near the center of the brain to alleviate motor disorders such as essential tremor.[2,3] Thermal ablation by FUS is an attractive modality as it allows therapeutic lesioning without holes in the skull, much less incision in the overlying scalp. Noninvasive thermal ablation may also be applied to disrupt other aberrant networks in the brain, such as those underlying psychiatric disorders[4] and chronic pain.[5] However, currently there are limitations to where in the brain temperature can be raised high enough for ablation. Another promising application of FUS has been in the ability to mechanically disrupt the blood–brain barrier (BBB). This occurs through the mechanical effects of FUS on intravascular microbubbles.[1,6]

The BBB is central to maintaining the homeostasis in the brain by its selective permeability and its role in neuro-immunology. An estimated 98% of all drugs do not enter the brain parenchyma to a significant extent due to the selectively permeable barrier imposed by the BBB.[7] Factors such as the size and hydrophilicity/lipophilicity determine the extent that the barrier is permeable to a molecule. It has also been theorized to be a substantial constraint on the release of DNA, proteins, exosomes from the brain parenchyma that could be useful in diagnosing and monitoring disease in the brain through peripheral blood samples, as in liquid biopsy.[8]

Use of FUS for either disrupting the BBB, or exerting mechanical or thermal forces on the target tissue, might improve the shedding of

---

[a] Division of Neurosurgery, Sunnybrook Health Sciences Centre, University of Toronto, 2075 Bayview Avenue, Toronto, Ontario, Canada; [b] Harquail Centre for Neuromodulation, Sunnybrook Health Sciences Centre, University of Toronto Canada, 2075 Bayview Avenue, Toronto, Ontario, Canada
* Corresponding author. Division of Neurosurgery, Sunnybrook Health Sciences Centre, University of Toronto, 2075 Bayview Avenue, Toronto, Ontario, Canada
E-mail address: nir.lipsman@utoronto.ca

Magn Reson Imaging Clin N Am 32 (2024) 699–704
https://doi.org/10.1016/j.mric.2024.04.006
1064-9689/24/© 2024 Elsevier Inc. All rights reserved, including those for text and data mining, AI training, and similar technologies.

biomarkers into blood. Data in animal studies and early data in clinical populations demonstrate a synergy between FUS and liquid biopsy techniques that holds the potential of transforming diagnosis of brain pathologies and early disease detection.[9–11]

PRINCIPLES OF FOCUSED ULTRASOUND

The principle of FUS is that multiple ultrasound beams are steered to converge onto a focal point within the body, with mechanical effects adding up at a converging target deep to the skin without affecting the intervening tissue. The main biological effects of FUS are thermal or mechanical.[1] These effects can be leveraged to ablate tumors, disrupt tissue, or enhance drug delivery, depending on the desired therapeutic outcome.

With thermal deposition, temperature increases above 60° Celsius can lead to coagulative necrosis. In this way, FUS has been clinical approved for the ablation of deep brain targets, prostate cancer, uterine fibroids, and bone tumors.[1] With the ability to efficiently deliver FUS across the intact skull, it was now possible to make precise, image-guided lesions noninvasively. During delivery, the process is monitored in real-time with MR thermometry, allowing prediction of the postprocedure lesion location and size. At the same time, with sub-lesional temperatures, a clinical effect can often be detected, particularly in readily observable functional symptoms like tremor. This gave clinicians measurable feedback to best determine the lesion location while mitigating risk of side effects.

At lower intensities, the mechanical effects of FUS can be augmented with intravenous microbubbles, an effect which has been harnessed to induce transient separation of endothelial cells composing and maintaining the low permeability of the BBB.[7] This has been shown to occur through both separation of tight junctions, reduction of expression of proteins composing tight junctions as well as reduced expression of drug efflux transporters, and an increase in transcellular processes like caveolar vesicle trafficking.[7,12,13] The initial extent of BBB opening and duration of time from FUS intervention to full restoration of BBB permeability are dependent on sonication parameters, particularly peak negative pressure.[14]

The disruption of the BBB by FUS concurrent with the delivery of intravenous therapies has been shown in hundreds of animal studies to improve the brain penetration of said therapies.[7] These results have been replicated in human studies through both imaging and biochemical assays.[15–17] FUS BBB opening appears effective at improving the brain penetrance of substances in systemic circulation. Evidence suggests that the window for drug delivery, or apparent half-time of BBB closure, is negatively related to the size of the therapeutic being delivered.[18] Nonetheless, successful delivery of large therapeutics has been repeatedly demonstrated in animal models,[7] with early data suggesting translation to human subjects.[15] While therapeutics above approximately 500 Da are often unable to cross the BBB,[19] FUS BBB opening has demonstrated success in delivering large molecules such as trastuzumab (150 kDa, or hydrodynamic diameter of ~10 nm)[15,20] as well as adenoviruses (20 nm) and liposomes (>200 nm).[7]

At the same time, it might be conceivable that because the BBB acts as a 2-way street, brain-derived endogenous markers might be able to transverse into the blood. Conventional blood-based cell-free DNA (cfDNA) assays intended for liquid biopsy in oncology have demonstrated high sensitivity for ctDNA detection in peripheral tumors with higher cfDNA concentration, but much lower sensitivity in glioma patients who also tend to have much lower blood cfDNA concentrations.[8] In clinic, CSF has increasingly been shown to be valuable in tracking the burden and evolution of disease.[21] However, this approach would require multiple lumbar punctures, which is more invasive and associated with low but not zero morbidity. In vivo, DNA is wound around histones assemblies called nucleosomes, and cfDNA exists predominantly as single nucleosome particles with a hydrodynamic diameter of 6 to 10 nm.[22] Thus, if success with drug delivery is a reliable indicator, FUS BBB opening is well positioned to liberate particles of this size from the brain parenchyma.

If FUS can enhance the shedding of biomarkers on the parenchymal side of the BBB, it is potentially powerful secondary benefit of the procedure that can be harnessed to improve the sensitivity as well as the spatial specificity of liquid biopsy techniques, improve personalized approach to medicine that has been shown to improve outcomes. Because the FUS beams can be steered, they can be targeted to different regions of the tumor and in theory selectively enrich biomarkers from a specific area. This is the ultimate goal of the FUS liquid biopsy approach.

ANIMAL STUDIES

Zhu and colleagues[9] first reported in 2018 on the feasibility of FUS with intravascular microbubbles to improve the sensitivity of nucleic acid biomarker detection. In this study, mice with an implanted enhanced green fluorescent protein (eGFP)-transduced glioma cell line underwent FUS BBB disruption at 3 grades of peak pressures (1.52, 2.74, and 3.53 MPa). Blood samples were collected 4 to 20 minutes after the interventions and through quantitative polymerase chain reaction (qPCR) analysis, circulating eGFP mRNA levels were found to be 1500 to 4800 times higher in animals treated with FUS relative to untreated controls. Additionally, it was reported that the lower pressure (1.48 MPa) appeared to be more efficient in releasing the biomarker than higher pressures.

Subsequent to this, a follow-up study was performed in mouse and pig xenograft models of using implanted human U87 glioblastoma cells carrying EGFRvIII and TERT C228 T mutations.[10] FUS BBB opening in these animals produced a robust increase in T1-weighted contrast-enhanced brain volume and a trend toward increased abundance of short-fragment cfDNA consistent with a mononucleosomal origin. Importantly, disruption of the BBB led to increased detection of tumor-derived EGFRvIII and TERT mutant DNA via digital-droplet PCR in blood collected 10 minutes after sonication in both mouse and pig models, with diagnostic sensitivity improved in both cases.[10] Optimization work reported in this study also suggests optimal detection of eGFP mRNA in transfected xenograft tumors at 10 minutes post-sonication, relative to later 30 and 60 min timepoints. Although microhemorrhage and a small number of apoptotic cells were observed, these were predominantly restricted to the sonicated tumor and their abundance did not differ significantly between the tumor and unsonicated brain parenchyma or control animals.[10] Thus, these differences may simply reflect tumor pathology rather than specific effects of FUS BBB disruption.

Other animal studies have expanded the scope of species, disease models, and biomarkers biopsied using FUS BBB opening. For example, FUS BBB opening in healthy pigs was able to increase concentrations of astrocyte-derived glial fibrillary acidic protein and oligodendrocyte-derived myelin basic protein approximately 2 to 4x without evidence of acute hemorrhage on T2*-weighted imaging or gross tissue damage upon histologic examination.[23] Similarly, FUS BBB opening at 0.68 MPa in transgenic mouse models of human tauopathies resulted in immediate post-FUS elevation of the ratio of phosphorylated tau to total tau, albeit with some microhemorrhages.[24] A subsequent experiment in the same study using 0.4 MPa FUS BBB opening detected elevated levels of neurofilament light (NfL) chain, a marker

of axonal degeneration, without microhemorrhage or other tissue damage apparent on histology.

CURRENT STATE IN CLINICAL STUDIES

Results from the animal studies provided the impetus for initial testing in human subjects. In a study investigating the safety and feasibility of combining MR-guided FUS to adjuvant temozolomide chemotherapy in patients after resection of their high-grade gliomas, blood samples were also collected as a secondary objective to confirm the preclinical findings. In these samples, the study found a 2 to 5 fold in circulating free DNA, and potentially enhancement of extracellular vesicles.[11] Additionally, we demonstrated a approximately 1.4 fold increase in the glial cell-derived protein S100β.

A phase I clinical trial was designed to specifically investigate this question. In this study, a portable neuronavigated FUS system was used to open the BBB in patients with suspected high-grade gliomas prior to their surgical resection (**Fig. 1A-D**).[25] Targeted sequencing using personalized mutation panels and digital droplet PCR measurements of TERT mutant cfDNA suggests enhanced systemic availability of tumor DNA after sonication.[11,25] Additionally, although longitudinal sample collection in this study demonstrated a significant individual variability in peak cfDNA concentration, significantly increased tumor variant, TERT mutant, and total cfDNA were observed at 10 and 30 min post-sonication in several patients suggesting a reasonably broad window for sampling.

Another multicenter study is currently ongoing using MR-guided FUS system to test whether the procedure can enhance cfDNA and ctDNA levels in patients with glioblastoma with tissues collected also at the time of surgery (NCT05383872). This study is an open-label design aiming to recruit 57 participants across numerous centers, with centralized sample processing. It is estimated to complete recruitment in early 2025.

In our institution's study of FUS BBB opening throughout the default mode network of patients with Alzheimer's disease, we demonstrated an increase in the neuronal axon-derived biomarker NfL chain after BBB disruption.[26] This is consistent with prior preclinical work at other institutions demonstrating increased GFAP in the blood of healthy pigs as well as increased circulating NfL chain in a transgenic murine tauopathy model after FUS BBB opening, both in the absence of gross parenchymal damage on histology.[23,24] Nonetheless, we did not observe increased levels of phosphorylated tau or amyloid-β species post-FUS versus pre-FUS BBB opening.

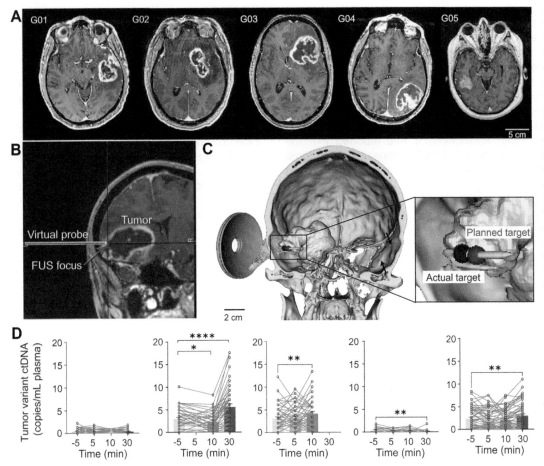

Fig. 1. (*A*) Contrast-enhanced T1-weighted structural imaging in 5 patients with high-grade gliomas who underwent neuronavigated FUS liquid biopsy prior to surgical resection. (*B*) Representative intraoperative neuronavigation showing FUS transducer aligned with a target within the tumor, near the enhancing margin. (*C*) Three-dimensional reconstruction of a representative patient's skull and tumor mass, with simulated focus of the FUS trajectory obtained by neuronavigation. (*D*) Profiling of plasma-derived circulating tumor DNA by personalized cfDNA assay informed by individual tumor genetics. *$p < .05$, **$p < .01$, ***$p < 0.001$, ****$p < .0001$. (Figures reproduced with modifications from Yuan et al., 2023[25] under a Creative Commons 4.0 license [http://creativecommons.org/licenses/by/4.0/].)

LIMITATIONS AND FUTURE DIRECTIONS

The rationale for the integration of FUS to liquid biopsy consists of both enhancing the biomarkers from pathologies behind the BBB and enriching the circulating biomarker of a spatially targeted region. In this way, one can conceive of sampling a specific tumor region that of interest such as areas of progression in previously treated tumors. Perhaps the detection of a new mutation would allow a patient the opportunity for novel targeted therapies. There have been numerous proof-of-concept studies in animal models. However, further advancement in this field is waiting for a clear demonstration of increased sensitivity and specificity of biomarker detection from blood samples taken after FUS. A major limitation has been the systematic collection of blood and tissue samples in device trials, where the device and technology itself are in their early testing phase. Nevertheless, a clinical trial currently under way with recruitment using the image-guided multiple transducer technology (NCT05383872) to address these questions. Another area of research is whether FUS can liberate brain parenchymal biomarkers into the cerebrospinal fluid, which has been shown to provide better signal-to-noise ratio than plasma samples for brain tumors.[27] As the integration of FUS into clinical care pathways improved, both in terms of lessened burden and proven efficacy of drug delivery, there will be opportunities to test its impact on circulating biomarkers. Understanding these relationships will allow us to circle back to using FUS for drug delivery, ultimately enhancing personalized medicine.

CLINICS CARE POINTS

- Focused ultrasound liquid biopsy is an emerging area of research currently in the clinical trial phase, and is currently not used in the clinical care setting.

REFERENCES

1. Meng Y, Hynynen K, Lipsman N. Applications of focused ultrasound in the brain: from thermoablation to drug delivery. Nat Rev Neurol 2021;17(1):7–22.
2. Elias WJ, Lipsman N, Ondo WG, et al. A Randomized Trial of Focused Ultrasound Thalamotomy for Essential Tremor. N Engl J Med 2016; 375(8):730–9.
3. Lipsman N, Schwartz ML, Huang Y, et al. MR-guided focused ultrasound thalamotomy for essential tremor: a proof-of-concept study. Lancet Neurol 2013;12(5):462–8.
4. Davidson B, Hamani C, Rabin JS, et al. Magnetic resonance-guided focused ultrasound capsulotomy for refractory obsessive compulsive disorder and major depressive disorder: clinical and imaging results from two phase I trials. Mol Psychiatr 2020; 25(9):1946–57.
5. Ahmed AK, Zhuo J, Gullapalli RP, et al. Focused Ultrasound Central Lateral Thalamotomy for the Treatment of Refractory Neuropathic Pain: Phase I Trial. Neurosurgery 2024;94(4):690.
6. Meng Y, Jones RM, Davidson B, et al. Technical Principles and Clinical Workflow of Transcranial MR-Guided Focused Ultrasound. Stereotact Funct Neurosurg 2021;99(4):329–42.
7. Meng Y, Pople CB, Lea-Banks H, et al. Safety and efficacy of focused ultrasound induced blood-brain barrier opening, an integrative review of animal and human studies. J Contr Release 2019;309: 25–36.
8. Bettegowda C, Sausen M, Leary RJ, et al. Detection of Circulating Tumor DNA in Early- and Late-Stage Human Malignancies. Sci Transl Med 2014;6(224): 224ra24.
9. Zhu L, Cheng G, Ye D, et al. Focused Ultrasound-enabled Brain Tumor Liquid Biopsy. Sci Rep 2018; 8(1):6553.
10. Pacia CP, Yuan J, Yue Y, et al. Sonobiopsy for minimally invasive, spatiotemporally-controlled, and sensitive detection of glioblastoma-derived circulating tumor DNA. Theranostics 2022;12(1):362–78.
11. Meng Y, Pople CB, Suppiah S, et al. MR-guided focused ultrasound liquid biopsy enriches circulating biomarkers in patients with brain tumors. Neuro Oncol 2021;23(10):1789–97.
12. Sheikov N, McDannold N, Sharma S, et al. Effect of Focused Ultrasound Applied With an Ultrasound Contrast Agent on the Tight Junctional Integrity of the Brain Microvascular Endothelium. Ultrasound Med Biol 2008;34(7):1093–104.
13. Cho H, Lee HY, Han M, et al. Localized Downregulation of P-glycoprotein by Focused Ultrasound and Microbubbles induced Blood-Brain Barrier Disruption in Rat Brain. Sci Rep 2016;6(1): 31201.
14. Chu PC, Chai WY, Tsai CH, et al. Focused Ultrasound-Induced Blood-Brain Barrier Opening: Association with Mechanical Index and Cavitation Index Analyzed by Dynamic Contrast-Enhanced Magnetic-Resonance Imaging. Sci Rep 2016;6: 33264.
15. Meng Y, Reilly RM, Pezo RC, et al. MR-guided focused ultrasound enhances delivery of trastuzumab to Her2-positive brain metastases. Sci Transl Med 2021;13(615):eabj4011.
16. Anastasiadis P, Gandhi D, Guo Y, et al. Localized blood–brain barrier opening in infiltrating gliomas with MRI-guided acoustic emissions–controlled focused ultrasound. Proc Natl Acad Sci USA 2021; 118(37):e2103280118.
17. Sonabend AM, Gould A, Amidei C, et al. Repeated blood–brain barrier opening with an implantable ultrasound device for delivery of albumin-bound paclitaxel in patients with recurrent glioblastoma: a phase 1 trial. Lancet Oncol 2023;24(5):509–22.
18. Marty B, Larrat B, Van Landeghem M, et al. Dynamic Study of Blood–Brain Barrier Closure after its Disruption using Ultrasound: A Quantitative Analysis. J Cereb Blood Flow Metab 2012;32(10): 1948–58.
19. Nance E, Pun SH, Saigal R, et al. Drug delivery to the central nervous system. Nat Rev Mater 2022; 7(4):314–31.
20. Ramos J, Vega JF, Cruz V, et al. Hydrodynamic and Electrophoretic Properties of Trastuzumab/HER2 Extracellular Domain Complexes as Revealed by Experimental Techniques and Computational Simulations. Int J Mol Sci 2019;20(5):1076.
21. Miller AM, Shah RH, Pentsova EI, et al. Tracking tumour evolution in glioma through liquid biopsies of cerebrospinal fluid. Nature 2019;565(7741): 654–8.
22. Banerjee A, Majumder P, Sanyal S, et al. The DNA intercalators ethidium bromide and propidium iodide also bind to core histones. FEBS Open Bio 2014;4:251–9.
23. Pacia CP, Zhu L, Yang Y, et al. Feasibility and safety of focused ultrasound-enabled liquid biopsy

in the brain of a porcine model. Sci Rep 2020; 10(1):7449.

24. Pacia CP, Yuan J, Yue Y, et al. Focused Ultrasound–mediated Liquid Biopsy in a Tauopathy Mouse Model. Radiology 2023;307(2):e220869.

25. Yuan J, Xu L, Chien CY, et al. First-in-human prospective trial of sonobiopsy in high-grade glioma patients using neuronavigation-guided focused ultrasound. npj Precis Onc 2023;7(1):92.

26. Meng Y, Goubran M, Rabin JS, et al. Blood–brain barrier opening of the default mode network in Alzheimer's disease with magnetic resonance-guided focused ultrasound. Brain 2023;146(3): 865–72.

27. Friedman JS, Hertz CAJ, Karajannis MA, et al. Tapping into the genome: the role of CSF ctDNA liquid biopsy in glioma. Neuro-Oncology Advances 2022; 4(Supplement_2):ii33–40.

Future Directions of MR-guided Focused Ultrasound

Dayton P. Grogan, MD[a], Timour Abduhalikov, BS[b], Neal F. Kassell, MD[c],
Shayan Moosa, MD[d],*

KEYWORDS

- MR-guided focused ultrasound (MRgFUS) • Neurologic disorders
- High-intensity focused ultrasound (HIFU) • Low-intensity focused ultrasound (LIFU) • Histotripsy

KEY POINTS

- MR-guided focused ultrasound (MRgFUS) presents a technologically advanced and minimally invasive modality of treating intracranial pathology with submillimeter accuracy. Novel technologies are being studied to improve targeting and predict treatment outcomes.
- Outside of thermal lesioning with MRgFUS, other modalities that are under investigation include histotripsy, targeted drug delivery, sonodynamic therapy, liquid biopsy, and neuromodulation.
- MRgFUS is currently approved for thermal lesioning in essential tremor and Parkinson's disease, although new research supports applications in neuro-oncology, neurodegenerative disease, epilepsy, and psychiatric disorders as well.

INTRODUCTION

The use of transcranial focused ultrasound (FUS) as a means of therapy is not a new concept. Two brothers, William and Francis Fry, demonstrated the ability to create brain lesions through a craniotomy using high-intensity focused ultrasound (HIFU) in the 1950s.[1] This was adapted by Lars Leksell who then designed a specially modified frame and transducer for intracranial HIFU lesioning.[2] However, progress stalled in these early stages of development due to limitations in imaging modalities and transcranial ultrasound delivery, which would be required for accurate and incisionless treatments. These hurdles were overcome in the 1990s when MR imaging technology, in addition to MR thermometry, provided the means by which clinicians could monitor lesioning effects of HIFU in real time. Other advancements that made transcranial ultrasound treatments

possible were the development of phased array transducers and phase-correction technology. The first coupling of these technologies for MR-guided focused ultrasound (MRgFUS) treatment of intracranial pathology became viable in the early 2000s. While MRgFUS is now an approved therapy for medication-refractory essential tremor (ET) and certain motor manifestations of Parkinson's disease (PD), research into a variety of FUS-related therapies for a wide array of pathologies is underway with promising initial results.[3,4] It is therefore the goal of this article to review the future of MRgFUS by examining potential advancements in its clinical technology and applications.

ADVANCEMENTS IN IMAGE GUIDANCE

While current therapies using MRgFUS hinge upon the combination of preoperative or intraoperative

[a] Department of Neurosurgery, University of Virginia Hospital, 1215 Lee Street, Charlottesville, VA 22903, USA;
[b] University of Virginia, School of Medicine, 1215 Lee Street, Charlottesville, VA 22903, USA; [c] Focused Ultrasound Foundation, 1230 Cedars Ct Suite 206, Charlottesville, VA 22903, USA; [d] Department of Neurosurgery, University of Virginia Hospital, PO Box 800212, Charlottesville, VA 22908, USA
* Corresponding author. Department of Neurosurgery, University of Virginia Hospital, PO Box 800212, Charlottesville, VA 22908.
E-mail address: sm4cf@uvahealth.org

Magn Reson Imaging Clin N Am 32 (2024) 705–715
https://doi.org/10.1016/j.mric.2024.02.004
1064-9689/24/© 2024 Elsevier Inc. All rights reserved.

MR imaging and real-time MR thermometry, advancements in these fundamental technologies may improve and widen the scope of transcranial FUS applications.

Targeting

Accurate targeting is essential for MRgFUS treatments. MR-guided targeting methods, particularly for treating tremor, have generally utilized indirect targeting from anatomic landmarks[5] seen on T1- or T2-weighted MR imaging scans. However, there are significant individual differences in brain anatomy that can contribute to targeting error.[6,7]

Current research into identification of sonication targets using diffusion tensor imaging (DTI) and known anatomic connectivity has allowed for a degree of personalized preoperative planning, although there is still a lack of consensus on the best tracts to model.[5,8] For example, DTI has been used to highlight specific target structures, such as the ventral intermediate nucleus of the thalamus (VIM), by better assessing the associated dentatorubrothalamic tract, medial lemniscus, and internal capsule.[9]

Another approach is aimed at targeting based on direct visualization of specific targets, which may be difficult with standard T1- and T2-weighted MR imaging protocols. Sequences, such as the Fast Gray Matter Acquisition T1 Inversion Recovery (FGATIR) and White Matter Attenuated Inversion Recovery, aim to nullify white matter signal and enhance target visualization.[10,11] Other similar sequences include susceptibility-weighted imaging and proton density mapping.[12,13] While none are universally used, FGATIR has become common practice with many MRgFUS centers as it provides significantly better visualization of specific targets compared to standard 3-T (3T) T1-or T2-weighted imaging and also reveals features not visible on other scan types, such as the internal lamina of the globus pallidus internus, fiber bundles of the internal capsule, and boundaries of the subthalamic nucleus (STN).[10] This improved resolution is largely due to its shorter inversion time compared to the standard cerebrospinal fluid-nulled magnetization-prepared rapid gradient echo sequence, leading to dark white matter and bright cerebrospinal fluid, as well as improved distinction between subcortical gray matter structures.[5]

Other improvements in imaging aim to increase targeting resolution via 7-T (7T) MR imaging.[5,14] The use of 7T MR imaging instead of the traditional 3T scans is under investigation to provide immense structural detail to further aid patient planning for surgeries and to demonstrate posttreatment lesions more fully. For instance, studies with 7T MR imaging have examined lesions in patients after receiving MRgFUS thalamotomy for essential tremor (ET) and have demonstrated a large involvement of the cerebellothalamic tract with successful lesioning and only minor involvement of the VIM.[5,15] Imaging with such high definition may provide further details into the role of specific white matter tracts while further detailing structural characteristics of new and existing therapeutic targets. In addition, 7T MR imaging can be combined with white matter null imaging for optimization of intrathalamic contrast and localization of the VIM.[5,16]

Finally, recent transcranial ultrasound delivery systems have moved beyond frame-based stereotactic MR imaging guidance, which requires head fixation that can be uncomfortable for patients. One example is the NaviFUS (NaviFUS Inc.) system that uses clinically available optical neuronavigation to guide the ultrasound delivery (Fig. 1).[17,18] Through personalized simulation of focal beam and skull attenuation along with optical neuronavigation, NaviFUS intraoperatively directs ultrasound energy precisely toward targeted brain regions.[18] This innovation has made transcranial delivery of low-intensity focused ultrasound (LIFU) easier and less time-consuming for a variety of applications, including blood–brain barrier (BBB) opening, drug delivery, sonodynamic therapy, and liquid biopsy.[17,19]

Lesion Prediction

The goal of imaging and thermometry coupling is to establish well-defined and repeatable criteria for creating a planned lesion with long-term therapeutic effects, while avoiding excessive delivery of energy and potential associated side effects.[20] Yet, the ability to predict the evolution of a lesion based on thermal dosages remains limited. The development of such models is limited by the use of single-slice, two-dimensional (2D) Fourier transform imaging, which is unable to provide three-dimensional (3D) topographic data and temporal evolution of the lesion volume.[20,21] To this end, 3D thermometry is a sought-after technological advancement in MRgFUS. Some researchers have used threshold-based thermoablation models to predict the 3D topography of the lesion and its evolution in the short-to-mid term (24 hours to 3 months after the treatment). This can be accomplished through the combination of 2D thermal dose maps into a volumetric lesion reconstruction.

True multiple-slice or volumetric techniques have been proposed using multi-slice echo-planar imaging (EPI).[21] Regular EPI is acquired using a

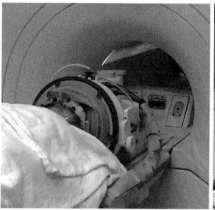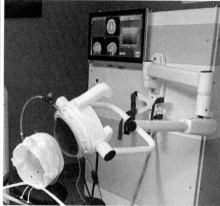

Fig. 1. NaviFUS system with STEALTH neuronavigation system (left), ultrasound transducer (bottom middle), holding arm (bottom right), and cabinet (right).

pulse sequence where multiple echoes of different phase steps are obtained with rephrasing gradients rather than repeated radiofrequency pulses. Thus, only one nuclear spin excitation is used per image, allowing for rapid image acquisition in a fraction of a second with excellent resolution.[22] Extension of this imaging technology to multiple slices simultaneously has been proposed for volumetric temperature monitoring.[21] This allows for focal spot localization in multiple dimensions with a single sonication and could eliminate the need for repeated localization sonications. Furthermore, it allows for tracking of the along-beam focal profile during treatment and could inform the user of temperature drift during sonication sessions.

Although still in development, the use of 3D thermometry and advanced imaging modalities may be useful in adapting machine learning to lesion prediction. Already, supervised machine learning algorithms have been used to predict treatment outcomes through postoperative imaging variables.[23] However, such methods have not been applied to real-time lesion creation where variables obtained from the ultrasound arrays and volumetric heating are used to predict lesion volume and subsequent physiologic effects.

ADVANCEMENTS IN ULTRASOUND DELIVERY

Historically, transcranial FUS has predominantly been delivered as a series of high-intensity beams that converge to result in thermal lesioning of targeted central nervous system (CNS) structures. This mechanism has driven the vast majority of its clinical indications thus far. However, novel usages of HIFU, as well as the incorporation of LIFU, have composed a large degree of investigation in recent years.

High-intensity Focused Ultrasound

The most well-known use of HIFU is for lesioning in the treatment of medically refractory ET and PD. HIFU targets remain isolated to central brain regions where the multiple acoustic beams are most optimally focused.[24] Unfortunately, lesioning of the cortex, the superficial subcortical areas, and regions close to the skull base is not currently possible with the current phased-array transducers in use.[24] Therefore, new HIFU ablative techniques, which are not based on thermal mechanisms, such as histotripsy, are being developed and tested in experimental settings to expand the treatment envelope.

While HIFU often achieves therapeutic benefit through thermal ablation, histotripsy involves a noninvasive, nonionizing, and nonthermal ablation methodology to mechanically destroy tissue through cavitation.[25] This underlying mechanism is unique and relies on mechanical disruption while minimizing heat output. In contrast to continuous or long bursts of ultrasound seen in traditional HIFU, histotripsy involves short ultrasound bursts with a low-duty cycle and high peak pressure amplitudes. This generates acoustic cavitation from endogenous gas inside of tissues, which reduces heat and results in localized intense strain that can fracture cells into acellular debris.[25–29] Ultrasound imaging is used to control and monitor histotripsy in real time, although there is recent research in MR-guided histotripsy. The properties of cavitation allow histotripsy to noninvasively remove biologic tissue from an individual.[25] This has allowed for an expansive list of clinical applications, such as with clot lysis and in liquid biopsies where cavitation results in liquification of the targeted tissue to an acellular homogenate that is then absorbed.[25,30,31]

Other techniques have utilized thermal effects of HIFU without generating lesions. Such an example is the role of HIFU in immunomodulation, which became a target of cancer-related research when it was realized that certain tumor types are associated with a reduced immune response.[32] For instance, the most common genetic alteration in glioblastoma multiforme (GBM) is loss of phosphatase and tensin homologue gene expression.[32–34] This leads to a decrease in tumor cell immunogencity by increasing anti-inflammatory cytokine release.[32,35] Working synergistically with genetic alterations is an associated tumor-induced microenvironment comprised of extracellular matrix and vascular networks, in addition to increased anti-inflammatory cytokines. This local environment promotes tumor growth and renders immune cells into a dysfunctional or inactive state.[36] FUS as a potential treatment modality displays multiple antitumor features and can alter the associated tumor microenvironment.[32,37] HIFU targeted at specific tumor regions generates tissue heating, resulting in mechanical stimulation and release of danger-associated molecular patterns that can stimulate immune response and infiltration of dendritic cells (DCs). Such bioeffects may alter depending on specific FUS parameters, including frequency, pressure, duty cycle, and treatment times. Once DCs infiltrate the tumor microenvironments, they migrate to the draining lymph system and present tumor-associated antigens to circulating T cells—essentially serving as an effective immunogenic vaccine.[38]

Low-intensity Focused Ultrasound

While the thermal attributes of HIFU provide a robust degree of therapeutic applications, research into LIFU has also proven fruitful in developing novel therapeutic advancements. Specifically, its use has been beneficial in the development of strategies for BBB opening and drug delivery, sonodynamic therapy, liquid biopsy, and neuromodulation.

LIFU, similar to HIFU, may induce cavitation via the combination of microbubbles injected into the patient.[39] A low-frequency transducer can be used to target a specific brain region and induce circulating microbubbles (MBs) to generate cavitation. Similar to histotripsy, this results in mechanical strain onto blood vessels and causes transient and reversible BBB opening. Moreover, the use of MBs in LIFU results in a greater degree of potential therapeutic benefits not strongly available to histotripsy. For instance, electrostatic interactions may be used to coat drugs onto the surface of MBs.[40] Others may be encapsulated by the MBs

through hydrophobic interactions. Thus, pharmaceutical agents can evade exogenous enzyme degradation and increase their availability.

This aspect of LIFU is similar to yet another termed sonodynamic therapy, which leads to molecular alterations into pharmaceutical agents that are selectively taken up by tumor cells to activate tumor-toxic properties.[38] One study by Sheehan and colleagues in 2020 analyzed the effect of 5-aminolevulinic acid hydrochloride (5-ALA) with MRgFUS on glioblastoma cells. 5-ALA, selectively taken up by glioma cells and currently used as a fluorescent marker of such cells in an intraoperative context, also has the added effect of metabolizing and generating reactive oxygen species when hit by ultrasound radiation, thus selectively sensitizing glioma tissue to MRgFUS.[38,41,42] This study demonstrated a reduction in cell viability and increased apoptosis in rat and human glioblastoma cell lines.[38]

LIFU, similar to HIFU, may induce a degree of tissue heating, although not to the degree required for tissue ablation. Yet, this mild, sublethal heating, when focused onto tumor tissue, has been shown to result in the release of miRNAs via increased circulation and vasodilation.[43,44] Released miRNA could potentially then be detected in general blood samples, thus providing a form of liquid biopsy that can be used to aid tumor diagnosis and subsequently provide a degree of molecular characterization.[45]

Low-intensity ultrasound has also been shown to reversibly modulate region-specific brain function.[46] A number of in vivo studies have demonstrated that LIFU possesses the potential to both enhance and suppress neuronal activity without any associated neuronal damage. Such properties show promise for treating a number of neurologic and psychiatric disorders and hold advantage over more invasive techniques of modulation such as deep brain stimulation (DBS).

EXPANSION OF TREATMENT INDICATIONS
Movement Disorders

MRgFUS has been Food and Drug Administration (FDA) approved for use in ET and PD, and additional research has focused on improving current protocols and investigating new targets of ablation. With regard to ET, the landmark clinical trial published by Elias and colleagues in 2016 demonstrated the safety and efficacy of unilateral thalamotomy in reducing unilateral hand tremor.[3] However, many patients with ET experience bilateral tremor. An initial phase II clinical trial performed by Iorio-Morin and colleagues has demonstrated that bilateral, MRgFUS thalamotomy has similar

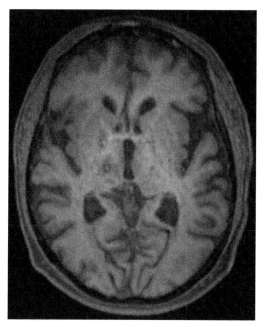

Fig. 2. MR imaging demonstrating bilateral, staged thalamotomies for ET. It is noted that the right lesion is larger than the right. This is because the right lesion is more recent, and lesion volume decreases with time.

safety and efficacy as unilateral treatment, though with reduction of tremor bilaterally.[47] For patients with bilateral symptoms and previous unilateral treatment, a clinical trial to evaluate safety and efficacy of returning for second contralateral treatment has recently been completed, and this treatment has been approved by the FDA since early 2023 (NCT04501484; **Fig. 2**).

Treatment of PD with MRgFUS has followed a similar course. Currently, FDA approval of MRgFUS for PD symptoms involves unilateral thalamotomy and pallidotomy, both demonstrating high- and long-term efficacy in reduction of tremor and dyskinesias, respectively.[48,49] A study by Martínez-Fernández and colleagues demonstrated improvement in motor symptoms following lesioning to the STN.[4] Moreover, additional clinical trials are underway evaluating safety and efficacy for both bilateral treatment protocols and new targets, including bilateral subthalamotomy and bilateral pallidothalamic tractotomy (NCT03964272 and NCT04728295).

Pain Disorders

Thermal lesioning using MRgFUS can be used to treat various pain disorders. The first related study was published in 2012 by Jeanmonod and colleagues in which the group determined the feasibility and safety of lesioning the posterior central lateral nucleus of the thalamus (CLT) for neuropathic pain in 12 patients.[50] A later study performed by Gallay and colleagues in 2023 expanded the study population and demonstrated efficacy and durability of CLT lesioning for general neuropathic pain, with a mean pain relief of 42% at 55 months follow-up.[51] The same group published a study in 2020 detailing CLT lesioning in 8 patients with trigeminal neuralgia. They found that at 1 year, patients reported a median pain relief of 75%.[52] Additionally, the 2023 study included subgroup analysis for 8 patients with trigeminal neuralgia, showing mean pain relief of 76% at a follow-up averaging 80 months.[51] A randomized, sham-controlled trial performed in 2023 by Ishaque and colleagues evaluated the efficacy of bilateral lesioning of the CLT in 10 patients with trigeminal neuropathic pain (5 underwent the treatment), finding no significant reduction in pain in the treatment group.[53] Additional studies with larger sample sizes of patients will help to elucidate the role of MRgFUS lesioning in the treatment of trigeminal neuralgia and neuropathic pain, and such studies are currently underway (NCT04579692). Another avenue for MRgFUS is the treatment of cancer-related pain. A current clinical trial is underway to determine the efficacy of mesencephalotomy for pain related to head and neck cancers (NCT03894553).

Psychiatric Disorders

MRgFUS also has potential for the treatment of psychiatric disorders. One study performed by Jung and colleagues in 2015 demonstrated that bilateral lesioning of the anterior limb of the internal capsule reduced symptoms of obsessive-compulsive disorder (OCD), depression, and anxiety in patients with treatment-refractory OCD. Four patients underwent the procedure and experienced decreased scores in the Yale-Brown obsessive-compulsive scale, Hamilton Anxiety Rating Scale, and Hamilton Depression Rating Scale in a 6 month follow-up period, with 2 patients achieving a "full response."[54]

Another study by Davidson and colleagues examined the safety profile, clinical response, and imaging correlates of bilateral anterior capsulotomy via MRgFUS in 12 patients—6 with refractory OCD and 6 with major depressive disorder.[55] Patients tolerated the procedures well and documented no serious adverse events. At follow-up, it was found that 4 of 6 and 2 of 6 responded to the treatment of OCD and major depressive disorder (MDD), respectively. At 6 months, additional PET imaging in 9 of 12 subjects demonstrated a widespread decrease in metabolism in both hemispheres bilaterally in addition to the right hippocampus, amygdala, and putamen—showing that capsulotomies generate both targeted and global changes in neural activity.

Brain Tumors

MRgFUS can aid in the delivery of drugs to the CNS parenchyma by transient and focal opening of the BBB. The mechanism of this action is multifaceted, likely a combination of shear forces of injected microbubbles vibrating with applied effects on endothelial cells, altering regulation on various transport proteins, and modulating function of ion channels.[56] As for the agents to be involved in this potential method of treatment, several preclinical studies have analyzed MRgFUS-mediated BBB opening coupled with administration of chemotherapeutic drugs and agents, including temozolomide, bevacizumab, trastuzumab, doxorubicin, carboplatin, mCD47, methotrexate, NK-92 (for HER2+ brain metastases), and immunoglobulins, assessing their ability to penetrate the CNS and alteration of survival and tumor metrics in animal models.[18,57–61] Currently, there are many ongoing clinical trials involving MRgFUS BBB opening and concurrent chemotherapeutic treatment, and most aim to characterize the safety and feasibility of BBB disruption with concurrent delivery of agents, such as temozolomide (NCT04998864). Others aim at comparing adjuvant and neoadjuvant administration of drugs like pembrolizumab with and without BBB disruption (NCT05879120).

In addition, another treatment method involving MRgFUS in glioma, termed sonodynamic therapy, involves combing ultrasound administration with substances that sensitize cells to the FUS treatment and is described earlier in further detail. There are at least 4 clinical trials ongoing for the use of sonodynamic therapy for GBM (NCT04845919; NCT06039709; NCT05370508; NCT05362409). Potential glioma therapies are now also being extended to pediatric patients and have been used in one case of a 5 year old girl found to have a pediatric diffuse intrinsic pontine glioma, which is being extended in a multi-patient trial.[62]

Liquid Biopsy

While mechanical disruption of the BBB can be used for drug delivery, this can also allow for noninvasive sampling of tumor areas via the vasculature. Two key studies have used this method in human trials. The first by Meng and colleagues demonstrated clinical feasibility of this technique by examining blood samples of 9 patients undergoing MRgFUS with adjuvant temozolomide for glioblastoma (NCT03616860).[63] Samples were obtained before and after sonication and compared with healthy individuals undergoing sonication alone. After-treatment samples demonstrated a greater than 2 fold increase in cfDNA. One patient with an IDH1 mutant tumor was found to have cfDNA-mutant copies of IDH1 in their blood after sonication, further indicating the potential for molecular typing via liquid biopsy. Another trial by Yuan and colleagues utilized a compact neuronavigation system to sonicate targeted tumor areas and induce cavitation to generate liquid biopsies in 5 patients.[19] Fig. 3 is derived from their work and demonstrates their study well (Fig. 3). Analysis of blood samples collected before and after sonication demonstrated an increase of 1.6 fold for mononucleosome cfDNA.[19]

Neurodegenerative Diseases

Similar to neuro-oncological indications for BBB opening, several agents and protocols have been studied in neurodegenerative diseases including Alzheimer's disease (AD), PD, and amyotrophic lateral sclerosis. While drug administration has only been studied in AD thus far, all 3 of the mentioned disease have undergone at least one proof-of-concept clinical trial demonstrating safe and durable BBB opening without concurrent drug administration.[64–68] For AD, one clinical trial performed by D'Haese and colleagues in 2020 demonstrated an average standardized uptake value ratio (SUVr) reduction in ^{18}F-Florbetaben, a PET β-amyloid imaging agent, of 5.05% ($\pm$2.76), indicating that simply BBB opening alone without therapeutic agents can assist in the treatment of AD. A recent study by Rezai and colleagues applied MR-guided LIFU with each of 6 monthly aducanumab infusions to temporarily open the BBB in 3 participants over a period of 6 months.[68] Results demonstrated a reduction in the level of Aβ proteins in regions treated with LIFU as compared to homologous regions in the contralateral hemisphere.

Epilepsy

Medication-refractory epilepsy has been treated with a variety of ablative and neuromodulatory techniques. Adaptations of FUS may add yet another modality for both treatment avenues. The anterior thalamic nucleus (ATN) has been used as an ablative targeted using MRgFUS.[69] One pilot-study adapting MRgFUS demonstrated the practical application of FUS for ATN ablation

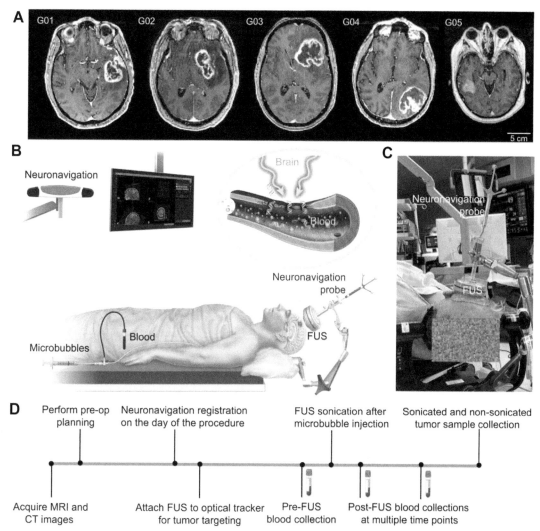

Fig. 3. (*A*) T1-weighted with contrast MR images before sonobiopsy of the 5 patients studied in the trial by Xu and colleagues. (*B*) Illustration of the neuronavigation-guided sonobiopsy setup. (*C*) FUS transducer coupled to the neuronavigation probe used during the sonobiopsy procedure. (D) Depiction of clinical workflow used in the trial. (*Data from* Yuan, J., Xu, L., Chien, CY. *et al.* First-in-human prospective trial of sonobiopsy in high-grade glioma patients using neuronavigation-guided focused ultrasound. *npj Precis. Onc.* **7**, 92 (2023). https://doi.org/10.1038/s41698-023-00448-y)

in 2 patients with treatment-refractory, focal onset epilepsy using the Exablate Neuro (Insightec) system.[70] Seizure frequency was reduced significantly in both patients, with one patient being seizure-free at 12 months. The second patient experienced a reduction in seizure frequency from 90 to 100 seizures per month to 3 to 6 seizures per month.

The use of ablative MRgFUS for epilepsy is not limited to the ATN but can be used in tumor-related epilepsy and may eventually be used in targeting novel areas of focus related to complex epileptic networks.[69,71,72] Another study by

Yamaguchi and colleagues recounts the use of MRgFUS for disconnection surgery in a 26 year old man with gelastic seizures related to a hypothalamic hamartoma.[71] After procedure results demonstrated complete seizure freedom over a 1 year follow-up period.

In addition, patients with epilepsy can potentially benefit from neuromodulation with MRgFUS. One study performed by Lin and colleagues in 2020 showed low-intensity MRgFUS in penicillin-induced epileptic nonhuman primate models reduced total seizure count and seizure rate 16 hours following the study procedure.[73] In addition, they showed a reduction in epileptiform membrane potentials in human brain biopsy samples from patients with temporal lobe epilepsy.[73] Moreover, navigation-guided LIFU using the NaviFUS system has been used in a recent pilot study in 6 individuals to induce neuromodulation, resulting in significant lower seizure frequency in 2 patients for 3 days posttreatment.[74]

SUMMARY

Therapeutic FUS has been developed over the past several decades and has only recently become clinically feasible due to advancements in imaging guidance and ultrasound delivery. Advancements in image guidance are making therapeutic FUS procedures safer, easier, more efficacious, and more durable. Recent and upcoming technological advancements in ultrasound delivery mechanisms are allowing clinicians to perform incisionless procedures to treat intracranial disease processes in new and exciting ways. Finally, the combination of these advancements in image guidance and ultrasound delivery will continue to significantly expand the indications for FUS treatments.

CLINICS CARE POINTS

- Advancements in FUS image guidance have made MRgFUS procedures safer, more durable, and more efficacious.
- Recent technological advancements in FUS delivery mechanisms allow for incisionless procedures to treat neuropathology that had not been amendable to FUS therapy in previous years.
- Such advancements have also expanded upon the therapies for pathology already being treated with FUS - such as Parkinson's Disease and Essential Tremot - allowing for greater degree of efficacy, bilateraly therapies, and adaptaion to other disease components.

DISCLOSURE

The authors describe no commercial or financial disclosures associated with this work.

REFERENCES

1. Fry W, Fry F. Fundamental neurological research and human neurosurgery using intense ultrasound. Phys Med 1958;37:148.

2. Jagannathan J, Sanghvi NT, Crum LA, et al. High-intensity focused ultrasound surgery of the brain: part 1—a historical perspective with modern applications. Neurosurgery 2009;64(2):201–11.

3. Elias WJ, Lipsman N, Ondo WG, et al. A randomized trial of focused ultrasound thalamotomy for essential tremor. N Engl J Med 2016;375(8):730–9.

4. Martínez-Fernández R, Máñez-Miró JU, Rodríguez-Rojas R, et al. Randomized trial of focused ultrasound subthalamotomy for Parkinson's disease. N Engl J Med 2020;383(26):2501–13.

5. Su JH, Choi EY, Tourdias T, et al. Improved Vim targeting for focused ultrasound ablation treatment of essential tremor: A probabilistic and patient-specific approach. Hum Brain Mapp 2020;41(17):4769–88.

6. Anthofer J, Steib K, Fellner C, et al. The variability of atlas-based targets in relation to surrounding major fibre tracts in thalamic deep brain stimulation. Acta Neurochir 2014;156:1497–504.

7. Brierley J, Beck E. The significance in human stereotactic brain surgery of individual variation in the diencephalon and globus pallidus. J Neurol Neurosurg Psychiatry 1959;22(4):287.

8. Akram H, Hariz M, Zrinzo L. Connectivity derived thalamic segmentation: Separating myth from reality. Neuroimage 2019;22:101758.

9. Krishna V, Sammartino F, Agrawal P, et al. Prospective tractography-based targeting for improved safety of focused ultrasound thalamotomy. Neurosurgery 2019;84(1):160–8.

10. Sudhyadhom A, Haq IU, Foote KD, et al. A high resolution and high contrast MRI for differentiation of subcortical structures for DBS targeting: the Fast Gray Matter Acquisition T1 Inversion Recovery (FGATIR). Neuroimage 2009;47:T44–52.

11. Vassal F, Coste J, Derost P, et al. Direct stereotactic targeting of the ventrointermediate nucleus of the thalamus based on anatomic 1.5-T MRI mapping with a white matter attenuated inversion recovery (WAIR) sequence. Brain Stimul 2012;5(4):625–33.

12. Abosch A, Yacoub E, Ugurbil K, et al. An assessment of current brain targets for deep brain stimulation surgery with susceptibility-weighted imaging at 7 tesla. Neurosurgery 2010;67(6):1745.

13. Spiegelmann R, Nissim O, Daniels D, et al. Stereotactic targeting of the ventrointermediate nucleus of the thalamus by direct visualization with high-field MRI. Stereotact Funct Neurosurg 2006;84(1):19–23.

14. Bluestein KT, Pitt D, Sammet S, et al. Detecting cortical lesions in multiple sclerosis at 7 T using white matter signal attenuation. Magn Reson Imaging 2012;30(7):907–15.

15. Purrer V, Upadhyay N, Borger V, et al. Lesions of the cerebello-thalamic tract rather than the ventral intermediate nucleus determine the outcome of focused

ultrasound therapy in essential tremor: A 3T and 7T MRI–study. Park Relat Disord 2021;91:105–8.

16. Saranathan M, Tourdias T, Bayram E, et al. Optimization of white-matter-nulled magnetization prepared rapid gradient echo (MP-RAGE) imaging. Magn Reson Med 2015;73(5):1786–94.

17. Chen K-T, Chai W-Y, Lin Y-J, et al. Neuronavigation-guided focused ultrasound for transcranial blood-brain barrier opening and immunostimulation in brain tumors. Sci Adv 2021;7(6):eabd0772.

18. Wei K-C, Tsai H-C, Lu Y-J, et al. Neuronavigation-guided focused ultrasound-induced blood-brain barrier opening: a preliminary study in swine. Am J Neuroradiol 2013;34(1):115–20.

19. Yuan J, Xu L, Chien C-Y, et al. First-in-human prospective trial of sonobiopsy in high-grade glioma patients using neuronavigation-guided focused ultrasound. NPJ Precis Oncol 2023;7(1):92.

20. López-Aguirre M, Caballero-Insaurriaga J, Urso D, et al. Lesion 3D modeling in transcranial MR-guided focused ultrasound thalamotomy. Magn Reson Imag 2021;80:71–80.

21. Marx M, Ghanouni P, Butts Pauly K. Specialized volumetric thermometry for improved guidance of mr g fus in brain. Magn Reson Med 2017;78(2):508–17.

22. Stehling MK, Turner R, Mansfield P. Echo-planar imaging: magnetic resonance imaging in a fraction of a second. Science 1991;254(5028):43–50.

23. Akpinar E, Bayrak O-C, Nadarajan C, et al. Role of machine learning algorithms in predicting the treatment outcome of uterine fibroids using high-intensity focused ultrasound ablation with an immediate non-perfused volume ratio of at least 90%. Eur Rev Med Pharmacol Sci 2022;26(22):8376–94.

24. Franzini A, Moosa S, Prada F, et al. Ultrasound ablation in neurosurgery: current clinical applications and future perspectives. Neurosurgery 2020;87(1):1–10.

25. Xu Z, Hall TL, Vlaisavljevich E, et al. Histotripsy: the first noninvasive, non-ionizing, non-thermal ablation technique based on ultrasound. Int J Hyperther 2021;38(1):561–75.

26. Movahed P, Kreider W, Maxwell AD, et al. Cavitation-induced damage of soft materials by focused ultrasound bursts: A fracture-based bubble dynamics model. J Acoust Soc Am 2016;140(2):1374–86.

27. Parsons JE, Cain CA, Abrams GD, et al. Pulsed cavitational ultrasound therapy for controlled tissue homogenization. Ultrasound Med Biol 2006;32(1):115–29.

28. Ter Haar GR. High intensity focused ultrasound for the treatment of tumors. Echocardiography 2001;18(4):317–22.

29. Khokhlova VA, Fowlkes JB, Roberts WW, et al. Histotripsy methods in mechanical disintegration of

tissue: Towards clinical applications. Int J Hyperther 2015;31(2):145–62.

30. Xu Z, Ludomirsky A, Eun LY, et al. Controlled ultrasound tissue erosion. IEEE Trans Ultrason Ferroelectrics Freq Control 2004;51(6):726–36.

31. Maxwell AD, Cain CA, Duryea AP, et al. Noninvasive thrombolysis using pulsed ultrasound cavitation therapy–histotripsy. Ultrasound Med Biol 2009;35(12):1982–94.

32. Cohen-Inbar O, Xu Z, Sheehan JP. Focused ultrasound-aided immunomodulation in glioblastoma multiforme: a therapeutic concept. Journal of Therapeutic Ultrasound 2016;4(1):1–9.

33. Aghi MK, Batchelor TT, Louis DN, et al. Decreased rate of infection in glioblastoma patients with allelic loss of chromosome 10q. Journal of Neuro-Oncology 2009;93:115–20.

34. Parsa AT, Waldron JS, Panner A, et al. Loss of tumor suppressor PTEN function increases B7-H1 expression and immunoresistance in glioma. Nat Med 2007;13(1):84–8.

35. Choe G, Horvath S, Cloughesy TF, et al. Analysis of the phosphatidylinositol 3′-kinase signaling pathway in glioblastoma patients in vivo. Cancer Res 2003;63(11):2742–6.

36. Gomez GG, Kruse CA. Mechanisms of malignant glioma immune resistance and sources of immunosuppression. Gene Ther Mol Biol 2006;10(A):133.

37. Joiner JB, Pylayeva-Gupta Y, Dayton PA. Focused ultrasound for immunomodulation of the tumor microenvironment. J Immunol 2020;205(9):2327–41.

38. Sheehan JP, Sheehan K, Sheehan D, et al. Investigation of the tumoricidal effects of sonodynamic therapy in malignant glioblastoma brain tumor models. Neurosurgery 2020;148(1):9–16.

39. Yan Y, Chen Y, Liu Z, et al. Brain delivery of curcumin through low-intensity ultrasound-induced blood–brain barrier opening via lipid-plga nanobubbles. Int J Nanomed 2021;16:7433–47.

40. Pysz MA, Willmann JK. Targeted Contrast-Enhanced Ultrasound: An Emerging Technology in Abdominal and Pelvic Imaging. Gastroenterology 2011;140(3):785–90.

41. Hadjipanayis CG, Widhalm G, Stummer W. What is the surgical benefit of utilizing 5-ALA for fluorescence-guided surgery of malignant gliomas? Neurosurgery 2015;77(5):663.

42. McHale AP, Callan JF, Nomikou N, et al. Sonodynamic therapy: concept, mechanism and application to cancer treatment. Therapeutic Ultrasound 2016;880:429–50.

43. Chevillet JR, Khokhlova TD, Giraldez MD, et al. Release of cell-free microRNA tumor biomarkers into the blood circulation with pulsed focused ultrasound: A noninvasive, anatomically localized, molecular liquid biopsy. Radiology 2017;283(1):158–67.

44. Kopechek JA, Kim H, McPherson DD, et al. Calibration of the 1-MHz Sonitron ultrasound system. Ultrasound Med Biol 2010;36(10):1762–6.

45. Hersh AM, Bhimreddy M, Weber-Levine C, et al. Applications of focused ultrasound for the treatment of glioblastoma: a new frontier. Cancers 2022;14(19):4920.

46. Baek H, Pahk KJ, Kim H. A review of low-intensity focused ultrasound for neuromodulation. Biomedical engineering letters 2017;7:135–42.

47. Iorio-Morin C, Yamamoto K, Sarica C, et al. Bilateral focused ultrasound thalamotomy for essential tremor (BEST-FUS phase 2 trial). Mov Disord 2021;36(11):2653–62.

48. Tewari AR, Grogan DP, Maragkos GA, et al. A New Era for Lesioning in Parkinson Disease. World neurosurgery 2023;179:236–7.

49. Chen T, Lin F, Cai G. Comparison of the efficacy of deep brain stimulation in different targets in improving gait in Parkinson's disease: a systematic review and Bayesian network meta-analysis. Front Hum Neurosci 2021;15:749722.

50. Jeanmonod D, Werner B, Morel A, et al. Transcranial magnetic resonance imaging–guided focused ultrasound: noninvasive central lateral thalamotomy for chronic neuropathic pain. Neurosurg Focus 2012;32(1):E1.

51. Gallay MN, Magara AE, Moser D, et al. Magnetic resonance–guided focused ultrasound central lateral thalamotomy against chronic and therapy-resistant neuropathic pain: retrospective long-term follow-up analysis of 63 interventions. J Neurosurg 2023;1(aop):1–10.

52. Gallay MN, Moser D, Jeanmonod D. MR-guided focused ultrasound central lateral thalamotomy for trigeminal neuralgia. Single center experience. Front Neurol 2020;11:271.

53. Ishaque M, Moosa S, Urban L, et al. Bilateral focused ultrasound medial thalamotomies for trigeminal neuropathic pain: a randomized controlled study. J Neurosurg 2023;1(aop):1–11.

54. Jung H, Kim S, Roh D, et al. Bilateral thermal capsulotomy with MR-guided focused ultrasound for patients with treatment-refractory obsessive-compulsive disorder: a proof-of-concept study. Mol Psychiatr 2015;20(10):1205–11.

55. Davidson B, Hamani C, Huang Y, et al. Magnetic resonance-guided focused ultrasound capsulotomy for treatment-resistant psychiatric disorders. Operative Neurosurgery 2020;19(6):741–9.

56. Thombre R, Mess G, Kempski Leadingham KM, et al. Towards standardization of the parameters for opening the blood–brain barrier with focused ultrasound to treat glioblastoma multiforme: A systematic review of the devices, animal models, and therapeutic compounds used in rodent tumor models. Front Oncol 2023;12:1072780.

57. Liu H-L, Huang C-Y, Chen J-Y, et al. Pharmacodynamic and therapeutic investigation of focused ultrasound-induced blood-brain barrier opening for enhanced temozolomide delivery in glioma treatment. PLoS One 2014;9(12):e114311.

58. Liu H-L, Hsu P-H, Lin C-Y, et al. Focused ultrasound enhances central nervous system delivery of bevacizumab for malignant glioma treatment. Radiology 2016;281(1):99–108.

59. Kobus T, Zervantonakis IK, Zhang Y, et al. Growth inhibition in a brain metastasis model by antibody delivery using focused ultrasound-mediated blood-brain barrier disruption. J Contr Release 2016;238:281–8.

60. Lin Y-L, Wu M-T, Yang F-Y. Pharmacokinetics of doxorubicin in glioblastoma multiforme following ultrasound-Induced blood-brain barrier disruption as determined by microdialysis. J Pharmaceut Biomed Anal 2018;149:482–7.

61. Sonabend AM, Gould A, Amidei C, et al. Repeated blood–brain barrier opening with an implantable ultrasound device for delivery of albumin-bound paclitaxel in patients with recurrent glioblastoma: a phase 1 trial. Lancet Oncol 2023;24(5):509–22.

62. Syed HR, Kilburn L, Fonseca A, et al. First-in-human sonodynamic therapy with ALA for pediatric diffuse intrinsic pontine glioma: a phase 1/2 study using low-intensity focused ultrasound. J Neuro Oncol 2023;162(2):449–51.

63. Meng Y, Pople CB, Suppiah S, et al. MR-guided focused ultrasound liquid biopsy enriches circulating biomarkers in patients with brain tumors. Neuro Oncol 2021;23(10):1789–97.

64. Rezai AR, Ranjan M, D'Haese P-F, et al. Noninvasive hippocampal blood– brain barrier opening in Alzheimer's disease with focused ultrasound. Proc Natl Acad Sci USA 2020;117(17):9180–2.

65. Mehta RI, Carpenter JS, Mehta RI, et al. Ultrasound-mediated blood–brain barrier opening uncovers an intracerebral perivenous fluid network in persons with Alzheimer's disease. Fluids Barriers CNS 2023;20(1):1–16.

66. Pineda-Pardo JA, Gasca-Salas C, Fernández-Rodríguez B, et al. Striatal Blood–Brain Barrier Opening in Parkinson's Disease Dementia: A Pilot Exploratory Study. Mov Disord 2022;37(10):2057–65.

67. Abrahao A, Meng Y, Llinas M, et al. First-in-human trial of blood–brain barrier opening in amyotrophic lateral sclerosis using MR-guided focused ultrasound. Nat Commun 2019;10(1):4373.

68. Rezai AR, D'Haese P-F, Finomore V, et al. Ultrasound Blood–Brain Barrier Opening and Aducanumab in Alzheimer's Disease. N Engl J Med 2024;390(1):55–62.

69. Cole ER, Grogan DP, Laxpati NG, et al. Evidence supporting deep brain stimulation of the medial

septum in the treatment of temporal lobe epilepsy. Epilepsia 2022;63(9):2192–213.

70. Krishna V, Mindel J, Sammartino F, et al. A phase 1 open-label trial evaluating focused ultrasound unilateral anterior thalamotomy for focal onset epilepsy. Epilepsia 2023;64(4):831–42.

71. Yamaguchi T, Hori T, Hori H, et al. Magnetic resonance–guided focused ultrasound ablation of hypothalamic hamartoma as a disconnection surgery: a case report. Acta Neurochir 2020;162:2513–7.

72. Grogan DP, Skelton HM, Fernandez AM, et al. The laterodorsal tegmentum and seizure regulation: Revisiting the evidence. J Neurosci Res 2023;101(2): 256–62.

73. Lin Z, Meng L, Zou J, et al. Non-invasive ultrasonic neuromodulation of neuronal excitability for treatment of epilepsy. Theranostics 2020;10(12):5514.

74. Lee CC, Chou CC, Hsiao FJ, et al. Pilot study of focused ultrasound for drug-resistant epilepsy. Epilepsia 2022;63(1):162–75.

UNITED STATES POSTAL SERVICE®

Statement of Ownership, Management, and Circulation
(All Periodicals Publications Except Requester Publications)

1. Publication Title	2. Publication Number	3. Filing Date
MAGNETIC RESONANCE IMAGING CLINICS OF NORTH AMERICA	011 – 909	9/18/2024

4. Issue Frequency	5. Number of Issues Published Annually	6. Annual Subscription Price
FEB, MAY, AUG, NOV	4	$420.00

7. Complete Mailing Address of Known Office of Publication (Not printer) (Street, city, county, state, and ZIP+4®)

ELSEVIER INC.
230 Park Avenue, Suite 800
New York, NY 10169

Contact Person
Malathi Samayan

Telephone (Include area code)
91-44-4299-4507

8. Complete Mailing Address of Headquarters or General Business Office of Publisher (Not printer)

ELSEVIER INC.
230 Park Avenue, Suite 800
New York, NY 10169

9. Full Names and Complete Mailing Addresses of Publisher, Editor, and Managing Editor (Do not leave blank)

Publisher (Name and complete mailing address)

DOLORES MELONI, ELSEVIER INC.
1600 JOHN F KENNEDY BLVD. SUITE 1800
PHILADELPHIA, PA 19103-2899

Editor (Name and complete mailing address)

JOHN VASSALLO, ELSEVIER INC.
1600 JOHN F KENNEDY BLVD. SUITE 1800
PHILADELPHIA, PA 19103-2899

Managing Editor (Name and complete mailing address)

PATRICK MANLEY, ELSEVIER INC.
1600 JOHN F KENNEDY BLVD. SUITE 1800
PHILADELPHIA, PA 19103-2899

10. Owner (Do not leave blank. If the publication is owned by a corporation, give the name and address of the corporation immediately followed by the names and addresses of all stockholders owning or holding 1 percent or more of the total amount of stock. If not owned by a corporation, give the names and addresses of the individual owners. If owned by a partnership or other unincorporated firm, give its name and address as well as those of each individual owner. If the publication is published by a nonprofit organization, give its name and address.)

Full Name	Complete Mailing Address
WHOLLY OWNED SUBSIDIARY OF REED/ELSEVIER, US HOLDINGS	1600 JOHN F KENNEDY BLVD. SUITE 1800 PHILADELPHIA, PA 19103-2899

11. Known Bondholders, Mortgagees, and Other Security Holders Owning or Holding 1 Percent or More of Total Amount of Bonds, Mortgages, or Other Securities. If none, check box. ▶ ☐ None

Full Name	Complete Mailing Address
N/A	

12. Tax Status (For completion by nonprofit organizations authorized to mail at nonprofit rates) (Check one)
The purpose, function, and nonprofit status of this organization and the exempt status for federal income tax purposes:
☒ Has Not Changed During Preceding 12 Months
☐ Has Changed During Preceding 12 Months (Publisher must submit explanation of change with this statement)

PS Form **3526**, July 2014 [Page 1 of 4 (see instructions page 4)] PSN: 7530-01-000-9931 PRIVACY NOTICE: See our privacy policy on www.usps.com.

---

13. Publication Title	14. Issue Date for Circulation Data Below
MAGNETIC RESONANCE IMAGING CLINICS OF NORTH AMERICA	MAY 2024

15. Extent and Nature of Circulation			Average No. Copies Each Issue During Preceding 12 Months	No. Copies of Single Issue Published Nearest to Filing Date
a. Total Number of Copies (Net press run)			363	322
b. Paid Circulation (By Mail and Outside the Mail)	(1)	Mailed Outside-County Paid Subscriptions Stated on PS Form 3541 (Include paid distribution above nominal rate, advertiser's proof copies, and exchange copies)	280	250
	(2)	Mailed In-County Paid Subscriptions Stated on PS Form 3541 (Include paid distribution above nominal rate, advertiser's proof copies, and exchange copies)	0	0
	(3)	Paid Distribution Outside the Mails Including Sales Through Dealers and Carriers, Street Vendors, Counter Sales, and Other Paid Distribution Outside USPS®	66	59
	(4)	Paid Distribution by Other Classes of Mail Through the USPS (e.g., First-Class Mail®)	0	0
c. Total Paid Distribution (Sum of 15b (1), (2), (3), and (4))		▶	346	309
d. Free or Nominal Rate Distribution (By Mail and Outside the Mail)	(1)	Free or Nominal Rate Outside-County Copies Included on PS Form 3541	17	13
	(2)	Free or Nominal Rate In-County Copies Included on PS Form 3541	0	0
	(3)	Free or Nominal Rate Copies Mailed at Other Classes Through the USPS (e.g., First-Class Mail)	0	0
	(4)	Free or Nominal Rate Distribution Outside the Mail (Carriers or other means)	0	0
e. Total Free or Nominal Rate Distribution (Sum of 15d (1), (2), (3) and (4))		▶	17	13
f. Total Distribution (Sum of 15c and 15e)		▶	363	322
g. Copies not Distributed (See Instructions to Publishers #4 (page #3))		▶	0	0
h. Total (Sum of 15f and g)		▶	363	322
i. Percent Paid (15c divided by 15f times 100)		▶	95.31%	95.96%

* If you are claiming electronic copies, go to line 16 on page 3. If you are not claiming electronic copies, skip to line 17 on page 3.

PS Form **3526**, July 2014 (Page 2 of 4)

16. Electronic Copy Circulation	Average No. Copies Each Issue During Preceding 12 Months	No. Copies of Single Issue Published Nearest to Filing Date
a. Paid Electronic Copies	▶	
b. Total Paid Print Copies (Line 15c) + Paid Electronic Copies (Line 16a)	▶	
c. Total Print Distribution (Line 15f) + Paid Electronic Copies (Line 16a)	▶	
d. Percent Paid (Both Print & Electronic Copies) (16b divided by 16c × 100)	▶	

☒ I certify that 50% of all my distributed copies (electronic and print) are paid above a nominal price.

17. Publication of Statement of Ownership

☒ If the publication is a general publication, publication of this statement is required. Will be printed in the **NOVEMBER 2024** issue of this publication. ☐ Publication not required.

18. Signature and Title of Editor, Publisher, Business Manager, or Owner

Malathi Samayan - Distribution Controller

Malathi Samayan

Date 9/18/2024

I certify that all information furnished on this form is true and complete. I understand that anyone who furnishes false or misleading information on this form or who omits material or information requested on the form may be subject to criminal sanctions (including fines and imprisonment) and/or civil sanctions (including civil penalties).

PS Form **3526**, July 2014 (Page 3 of 4) PRIVACY NOTICE: See our privacy policy on www.usps.com

Moving?

Make sure your subscription moves with you!

To notify us of your new address, find your **Clinics Account Number** (located on your mailing label above your name), and contact customer service at:

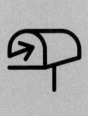

Email: journalscustomerservice-usa@elsevier.com

800-654-2452 (subscribers in the U.S. & Canada)
314-447-8871 (subscribers outside of the U.S. & Canada)

Fax number: 314-447-8029

Elsevier Health Sciences Division
Subscription Customer Service
3251 Riverport Lane
Maryland Heights, MO 63043

ELSEVIER

Printed and bound by CPI Group (UK) Ltd, Croydon, CR0 4YY

08/05/2025

01864750-0016